O C L
OXFORD CARDIOLOGY LIBRARY

Hypertension

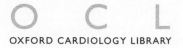

OXFORD CARDIOLOGY LIBRARY

Hypertension

THIRD EDITION

Edited by

Sunil K. Nadar

Senior Consultant Cardiologist, Sultan Qaboos University
Hospital, Muscat, Oman

Gregory Y. H. Lip

Price-Evans Chair of Cardiovascular Medicine, University of
Liverpool, UK; National Institute for Health Research (NIHR)
Senior Investigator; Consultant Cardiologist (Hon), Liverpool
Heart & Chest Hospital NHS Trust, Liverpool, UK

OXFORD
UNIVERSITY PRESS

OXFORD
UNIVERSITY PRESS

Great Clarendon Street, Oxford, OX2 6DP,
United Kingdom

Oxford University Press is a department of the University of Oxford.
It furthers the University's objective of excellence in research, scholarship,
and education by publishing worldwide. Oxford is a registered trade mark of
Oxford University Press in the UK and in certain other countries

First Edition published in 2009
Second Edition published in 2015
Third Edition published in 2023

Impression: 1

Published in the United States of America by Oxford University Press
198 Madison Avenue, New York, NY 10016, United States of America

British Library Cataloguing in Publication Data

Data available

Library of Congress Control Number: 2022941530

ISBN 978–0–19–887067–8

DOI: 10.1093/med/9780198870678.001.0001

Printed and bound by
CPI Group (UK) Ltd, Croydon, CR0 4YY

Acknowledgement to contributors of previous editions

The editors would like to thank the authors of the first and second editions whose excellent text and contributions have been continued into this third edition:

Mehmood Sadiq Butt
Girish Dwivedi
Shridar Dwivedi
Deepak Goyal
Pravin Jha
V. J. Karthikeyan
Mohammed Khan
Ayush Khurana
John Kurien
Rajesh Nambiar
Vasudevan A. Raghavan
Kully Sandhu
Jaspal Taggar
Viji Samuel Thomson
Timothy Watson
Shamil Yusuf

Contents

Contributors

Sarah Ahmad, Nephrology Fellow, Renal-Electrolyte and Hypertension Division, Department of Medicine, Perelman School of Medicine, University of Pennsylvania, Philadelphia, PA, USA

Asangaedem Akpan, Consultant Geriatrician, Liverpool University Hospitals NHS Foundation Trust, Liverpool, UK; Visiting Professor, University of Cumbria, Carlisle, UK; Honorary Associate Professor, University of Liverpool, Liverpool, UK; Ageing Specialty Research Group Lead, CRN NWC, Liverpool, UK

Hatim Al-Lawati, Senior Consultant Cardiologist, Department of Medicine, Sultan Qaboos University Hospital, Muscat, Oman

Mohammed Najeeb Al-Rawahi, Consultant Cardiac Electrophysiologist, Sultan Qaboos University Hospital, Muscat, Oman; Department of Cardiology, National Heart Center, Muscat, Oman

Hassan Al-Riyami, Head Nurse Cardiac Catheter Lab and Interventional Radiology, Directorate of Nursing, Sultan Qaboos University Hospital, Muscat, Oman

Benjamin J. R. Buckley, Research Fellow, Liverpool Centre for Cardiovascular Science, University of Liverpool and Liverpool Heart and Chest Hospital, Liverpool, UK

Jordana B. Cohen, Assistant Professor of Medicine and Epidemiology, Renal-Electrolyte and Hypertension Division, Center for Clinical Epidemiology and Biostatistics, Perelman School of Medicine, University of Pennsylvania, Philadelphia, PA, USA

Daniel J. Cuthbertson, Acute Medicine Consultant at University Hospital Aintree, Liverpool, UK, and Reader and Honorary Consultant Physician in the Department of Cardiovascular and Metabolic Medicine at the University of Liverpool

Christian Delles, Professor of Cardiovascular Prevention and Honorary Consultant Physician, School of Cardiovascular and Metabolic Health, University of Glasgow, Glasgow, UK

Stephanie J. Finnie, Trust Grade Doctor, Department of Medicine, Royal Liverpool University Hospital, Liverpool, UK

Harsh Goel, Consultant Physician, Department of Medicine, St Luke's University Hospital, Bethlehem, PA, USA; Associate Professor of Medicine, Lewis Katz School of Medicine, Temple University, Philadelphia, PA, USA

Arunodaya R. Gujjar, Professor of Neurology, Department of Medicine (Neurology), College of Medicine and Health Sciences, Sultan Qaboos University, Muscat, Oman

Stephanie L. Harrison, Lecturer, Liverpool Centre for Cardiovascular Science, University of Liverpool, Liverpool, UK

James Hatherley, Department of Medicine, Liverpool University Hospital Foundation Trust, Liverpool, UK

Vikas Kapil, Senior Lecturer and Consultant Physician, Clinical Pharmacology and Cardiovascular Medicine, Barts BP Centre of Excellence, St Bartholomew's Hospital, Barts Health NHS Trust, London, UK; Centre for Cardiovascular Medicine and Devices, William Harvey Research Institute, Queen Mary University, London, UK

Ashish Kumar, Consultant Hospitalist, Department of Medicine, Wellspan York Hospital, York, PA, USA; Clinical Assistant Professor of Medicine, Sidney Kimmel Medical College at Thomas Jefferson University, Philadelphia, PA, USA

Deirdre A. Lane, Professor of Cardiovascular Health, Liverpool Centre for Cardiovascular Science, University of Liverpool and Liverpool Heart and Chest Hospital, Liverpool, UK; Aalborg Thrombosis Research Unit, Department of Clinical Medicine, Aalborg University, Aalborg, Denmark

Chim C. Lang, Head, Division of Molecular and Clinical Medicine, School of Medicine, University of Dundee, Dundee, UK; Editor-in-Chief, *Cardiovascular Therapeutics*, Chairman–Heart Failure Working Group, Managed Clinical Network for CHD, Dundee, UK

Gregory Y. H. Lip, Price-Evans Chair of Cardiovascular Medicine, University of Liverpool, UK; National Institute for Health Research (NIHR) Senior Investigator; Consultant Cardiologist (Hon), Liverpool Heart & Chest Hospital NHS Trust, Liverpool, UK

Peck Lin Lip, Consultant Ophthalmologist (Medical Retina Specialist), Honorary Senior Lecturer, University of Birmingham, Birmingham and Midland Eye Centre, Sandwell and West Birmingham NHS Hospitals Trust, Birmingham, UK

Stephanie Lip, Specialist Registrar in Clinical Pharmacology and Therapeutics and General Internal Medicine, Queen Elizabeth University Hospital, Glasgow, UK

Chen Liu, Professor of Cardiology, Department of Cardiology, the First Affiliated Hospital of Sun Yat-Sen University, Guangzhou, Guangdong, China

Sheon Mary, Research Associate, School of Cardiovascular and Metabolic Health, BHF Glasgow Cardiovascular Research Centre, University of Glasgow, Glasgow, UK

Ify R. Mordi, Clinical Senior Lecturer and Consultant Cardiologist, University of Dundee and Ninewells Hospital and Medical School, Dundee, UK

Sunil K. Nadar, Senior Consultant Cardiologist, Department of Medicine, Sultan Qaboos University Hospital, Muscat, Oman

Sandosh Padmanabhan, Professor of Cardiovascular Genomics and Therapeutics, Institute of Cardiovascular and Medical Sciences, University of Glasgow, Glasgow, UK

Shankar Patil, Specialist Registrar, Leeds Teaching Hospitals NHS Trust, Leeds, UK

Giacomo Rossitto, Institute of Cardiovascular and Medical Sciences, BHF Glasgow Cardiovascular Research Centre, University of Glasgow, Glasgow, UK; Dipartimento di Medicina, DIMED, Università degli Studi di Padova, Padova, Italy

Thomas Salmon, Internal Medical Trainee, Warrington and Halton Teaching Hospitals NHS Foundation Trust, Warrington, UK

Rajiv Sankaranarayan, Heart Failure Clinical Lead (Aintree University Hospital and Community), Consultant Cardiologist, NIHR Research Scholar and Honorary Clinical Lecturer (University of Liverpool), Liverpool Centre for Cardiovascular Science, Liverpool University Hospitals NHS Foundation Trust, Liverpool, UK

Alena Shantsila, Tenure Track Fellow, Cardiovascular & Metabolic Medicine, University of Liverpool, Liverpool, UK

James P. Sheppard, University Research Lecturer, Wellcome Trust/Royal Society Sir Henry Dale Fellow, Nuffield Department of Primary Care Health Sciences, University of Oxford, Radcliffe Primary Care, Radcliffe Observatory Quarter, Oxford, UK

Gurbhej Singh, Assistant Professor of Cardiology, Dayanand Medical College and Hospital (Unit Hero DMC Heart Institute), Ludhiana, India

Gurpreet Singh Wander, Professor and Head of Cardiology, Dayanand Medical College and Hospital (Unit Hero DMC Heart Institute), Ludhiana, India

Jan A. Staessen, Professor Emeritus, Studies Coordinating Centre, Research Unit Hypertension and Cardiovascular Epidemiology, KU Leuven Department of Cardiovascular Diseases, University of Leuven, Campus Sint Rafaël, Kapucijnenvoer, Leuven, Belgium; Research Institute Alliance for the Promotion of Preventive Medicine, Mechelen, Belgium

Michael Stowasser, Director, Hypertension Unit, Princess Alexandra Hospital, Director, Endocrine Hypertension Research Centre, University of Queensland Diamantina Institute, Brisbane, Australia

Muzahir Tayebjee, Consultant Cardiologist, Leeds Teaching Hospitals NHS Trust, Leeds, UK

Gloria Valdés, Professor Emeritus, Departamento de Nefrología, Facultad de Medicina, Pontificia Universidad Católica, Santiago, Chile

Fang-Fei Wei, Associate Professor, Research Unit Hypertension and Cardiovascular Epidemiology, KU Leuven Department of Cardiovascular Diseases, University of Leuven, Leuven, Belgium; Department of Cardiology, the First Affiliated Hospital of Sun Yat-Sen University, Guangzhou, Guangdong, China

Martin Wolley, Consultant Nephrologist, Department of Renal Medicine, Royal Brisbane and Women's Hospital, Hypertension Unit, Princess Alexandra Hospital, University of Queensland, Brisbane, Australia

Yuichiro Yano, Associate Professor, Duke University School of Medicine, Durham, NC, USA; Vice Director, Center for Novel and Exploratory Clinical Trials, Associate Professor, Yokohama City University, Yokohama, Japan

List of symbols and abbreviations

ABC	Ascertaining Barriers to Compliance
ABPM	ambulatory blood pressure measurement/monitoring
ACC	American College of Cardiology
ACCORD	The Action to Control Cardiovascular Risk in Diabetes
ACE	angiotensin-converting enzyme
ACE2	angiotensin-converting enzyme 2
ACEI	angiotensin-converting enzyme inhibitor
ACTH	adrenocorticotrophic hormone
ADA	American Diabetes Association
ADVANCE	Action in Diabetes and Vascular Disease-PreterAx and DiamicroN Controlled Evaluation
AF	atrial fibrillation
AHA	American Heart Association
AHI	Apnoea-Hypopnoea Index
ALLHAT	Antihypertensive and Lipid-Lowering Treatment to Prevent Heart Attack Trial
ALTITUDE	The Aliskiren Trial in Type 2 Diabetes Using Cardiorenal Endpoints
AMI	acute myocardial infarction
ANP	atrial natriuretic peptide
AOBP	automated office blood pressure
APA	aminopeptidase A
ARA2	angiotensin II receptor antagonist
ARB	angiotensin receptor blocker
ARIC	Atherosclerosis Risk in Communities
ARNI	angiotensin receptor–neprilysin inhibitor
ASCOT	Anglo-Scandinavian Cardiac Outcomes Trial
ASCOT-BPLA	Anglo-Scandinavian Cardiac Outcomes Trial-Blood Pressure Lowering Arm
ASCVD	atherosclerotic cardiovascular disease
ASE	American Society of Echocardiography
ASPIRANT	Addition of spironolactone in patients with resistant arterial hypertension

ASTRAL	Angioplasty and Stent for Renal Artery Lesions
ATP	adenosine triphosphate
AT-R1	angiotensin type 1 receptor
AV	arteriovenous
BIHS	British and Irish Hypertension Society
BMI	body mass index
BNP	brain natriuretic peptide
BP	blood pressure
Ca^{2+}	calcium
CAA	cerebral amyloid angiopathy
CAFE	Conduit Artery Functional Endpoint
cAMP	cyclic adenosine monophosphate
CCB	calcium channel blocker
CCS	Canadian Cardiovascular Society
cGMP	cyclic guanosine monophosphate
CHARM	Candesartan in Heart Reduction in Mortality and Morbidity
CHD	coronary heart disease
CHF	congestive heart failure
CI	confidence interval
CIBIS-II	Cardiac Insufficiency Bisoprolol Study II
CKD	chronic kidney disease
Cl^-	chloride
CMB	cerebral micro-bleed
CNS	central nervous system
COMMIT/CCS-2	Clopidogrel and Metoprolol in Myocardial Infarction Trial/Second Chinese Cardiac Study
CONVINCE	Controlled ONset Verapamil INvestigation of Cardiovascular Endpoints
CORAL	Cardiovascular Outcomes in Renal Atherosclerotic Lesions
CSVD	cerebral small vessel disease
CT	computed tomography
CVD	cardiovascular disease
DALY	disability-adjusted life year
DASH	Dietary Approaches to Stop Hypertension

DBP	diastolic blood pressure
DENERHTN	The Renal Denervation for Hypertension trial
DETAIL	Diabetics Exposed to Telmisartan And enalaprIL
DOAC	direct oral anticoagulant
DOC	deoxycorticosterone
DPP-4	dipeptidyl peptidase 4
ECG	electrocardiogram/electrocardiography
EF	ejection fraction
eGFR	estimated glomerular filtration rate
ELITE	Evaluation of Losartan In The Elderly
EMPHASIS-HF	The Eplerenone in Mild Patients Hospitalization and Survival Study in Heart Failure trial
ENaC	epithelial sodium channel
EPHESUS	Eplerenone Post–Acute Myocardial Infarction Heart Failure Efficacy and Survival Study
ESC	European Society of Cardiology
ESCVI	European Society of Cardiovascular Imaging
ESH	European Society of Hypertension
ESS	Epworth Sleepiness Scale
EUROPA	European trial On Reduction of Cardiac Events with Perindopril in Stable Coronary Artery Disease
EVA	Epidemiology of Vascular Ageing
EVT	extravillous trophoblast
FIDELIO-DKD	The Finerenone in Reducing Kidney Failure and Disease Progression in Diabetic Kidney Disease trial
FLAIR	fluid-attenuated inversion recovery
FRESH	Firibastat in Treatment-resistant Hypertension
FMD	fibromuscular dysplasia
GBD	Global Burden of Disease
GEMINI	Glycemic Effect of Diabetes Mellitus: Carvedilol-Metoprolol Comparison In Hypertensives
GFR	glomerular filtration rate
GH	growth hormone
GLP-1	glucagon-like peptide 1
GUSTO-1	Global Utilization of Streptokinase and Tissue Plasminogen Activator for Occluded Coronary Arteries

GWAS	genome-wide association studies
HAAS	Honolulu-Asia Aging Study
HbA1c	glycated haemoglobin
HBPM	home blood pressure monitoring
HDL	high-density lipoprotein
HDP	hypertensive disorders of pregnancy
HELLP	haemolysis, elevated liver enzymes, low platelets
HFpEF	heart failure with preserved ejection fraction
HFrEF	heart failure with reduced ejection fraction
HMOD	hypertension-mediated organ damage
HOPE	Heart Outcomes Prevention Evaluation
HOPE-3	Heart Outcomes Prevention Evaluation-3
HOT	Hypertension Optimal Treatment
HR	hazard ratio
HYVET	Hypertension in the Very Elderly Trial
ICH	intracerebral haemorrhage
IGF-1	insulin-like growth factor 1
IL-6	interleukin 6
INSIGHT	International Nifedipine GITS Study of Intervention as a Goal in Hypertension Treatment
INSPiRED	AdenosINe Sestamibi Post-InfaRction Evaluation trial
INTERMAP	International Study of Macro- and Micro-nutrients and Blood Pressure
INTERSALT	The International study of Salt and Blood pressure
INVEST	International Verapamil Trandolapril Study
ISA	intrinsic sympathomimetic activity
ISH	International Society of Hypertension
ISIS-1	First International Study of Infarct Survival
ISSHP	International Society for the Study of Hypertension in Pregnancy
JNC-7	Seventh Report of the Joint National Committee on Prevention, Detection, Evaluation, and Treatment of High Blood Pressure
K^+	potassium
LA	left atrial/atrium
LDL	low-density lipoprotein

LIFE	Losartan Intervention for Endpoint reduction in hypertension
LIVE	Left Ventricular Hypertrophy Regression, Indapamide Versus Enalapril
LV	left ventricular
LVEDD	left ventricular end-diastolic diameter
LVEF	left ventricular ejection fraction
LVH	left ventricular hypertrophy
MARVAL	Microalbuminuria Reduction with VALsartan
MCI	minimal (mild) cognitive impairment
MEN	multiple endocrine neoplasia
MERIT-HF	Metoprolol CR/XL Randomised Intervention Trial in Congestive Heart Failure
MIAMI	Metoprolol In Acute Myocardial Infarction
MINISAL-SIIA	Ministero della Salute
MMAS-8	eight-item Morisky Medication Adherence Scale
MRA	mineralocorticoid receptor antagonist
MRC	Medical Research Council
MRFIT	Multiple Risk Factor Interventional Trial
MRI	magnetic resonance imaging
Na^+	sodium
NHS	National Health Service
NICE	National Institute for Health and Care Excellence
NO	nitric oxide
NORDIL	NORdic DILtiazem
NPRA	natriuretic peptide receptor agonist
OAT	organic acid transporter
ONTARGET	Ongoing Telmisartan Alone and in Combination With Ramipril Global Endpoint Trial
OPTIMAAL	OPtimal Trial in Myocardial Infarction with the Angiotensin II Antagonist Losartan
OSA	obstructive sleep apnoea
PARADIGM-HF	Prospective comparison of Angiotensin Receptor-neprilysin inhibitor (ARNI) with Angiotensin converting enzyme inhibitor (ACEI) to Determine Impact on Global Mortality and morbidity in Heart Failure

PARADISE-MI	Prospective ARNI vs ACE Inhibitor Trial to Determine Superiority in Reducing Heart Failure Events After MI
PARAGON-HF	Prospective Comparison of ARNI with ARB Global Outcomes in HF with Preserved Ejection Fraction
PARAMETER	Prospective Comparison of Angiotensin Receptor Neprilysin Inhibitor With Angiotensin Receptor Blocker Measuring Arterial Stiffness in the Elderly
PATHWAY-2	Prevention and Treatment of Hypertension with Algorithm based Therapy-2 trial
PE	pre-eclampsia
PEACE	Prevention of Events with Angiotensin-Converting Enzyme Inhibition
PET	positron emission tomography
PlGF	placental growth factor
PRA	plasma renin activity
PRESERVE	Prospective Randomized Enalapril Study Evaluating Regression of Ventricular Enlargement
PREVER-Prevention	Prevention of Hypertension in Patients with Pre-hypertension
PROGRESS	Perindopril Protection Against Recurrent Stroke Study
PROSPER	Pravastatin in Elderly Individuals at Risk of Vascular Disease
PTH	parathyroid hormone
PTWD	posterior wall thickness
PVD	peripheral vascular disease
RAAS	renin–angiotensin–aldosterone system
RADIANCE SOLO	A Study of the ReCor Medical Paradise System in Clinical Hypertension
RADIANCE TRIO	A Study of the ReCor Medical Paradise System in Clinical Hypertension
RALES	randomized aldactone evaluation study
RAS	renal artery stenosis
RAS	renin–angiotensin system
RCT	randomized controlled trial
RF	radiofrequency
RR	relative risk
rtPA	recombinant tissue plasminogen activator
RVH	renovascular hypertension

RVO	retinal vein occlusion
RWT	relative wall thickness
SBP	systolic blood pressure
SCAT	Simvastatin/Enalapril Coronary Atherosclerosis
SCOPE	Study on Cognition and Prognosis in the Elderly
SCORE	Systematic Coronary Risk Evaluation
SD	standard deviation
SEAMS	Self-efficacy for Appropriate Medication Use
sEH	soluble epoxide hydrolase
SGA	small-for-gestational-age
SGLT	sodium–glucose co-transporter
SGLT-2	sodium–glucose co-transporter-2
SHEP	Systolic Hypertension in the Elderly Program
SITS-ISTR	Safe Implementation of Thrombolysis in Stroke International Stroke Thrombolysis Register
SOLVD	Studies of Left Ventricular Dysfunction
SPAF-III	Stroke Prevention in Atrial Fibrillation III
SPRINT	Systolic Blood Pressure Intervention Trial
STOP-Hypertension	Swedish Trial in Old Patients with Hypertension
SWI	susceptibility-weighted image
SWTD	septal wall thickness
SYMPLICITY HTN-1	Renal sympathetic denervation in patients with treatment-resistant hypertension
Syst-China	Systolic Hypertension in the Elderly: Chinese trial
Syst-Eur	Systolic Hypertension in Europe
T2D	type 2 diabetes
TARGET	Telmisartan Alone and in Combination with Ramipril Global Endpoint Trial
TIA	transient ischaemic attack
TIMI-2B	Thrombolysis In Myocardial Infraction trial, phase II-B
TNF-α	tumour necrosis factor alpha
TOAST	Trial of ORG 10172 in Acute Stroke Treatment
TONE	Trial of Non-pharmacologic Intervention in the Elderly
TRACE	Trandolapril Cardiac Evaluation
TRANSCEND	Telmisartan Randomised Assessment Study in ACE Intolerant Subjects With Cardiovascular Disease
TSH	thyroid-stimulating hormone

UACR	urine albumin:creatinine ratio
UKPDS	UK Prospective Diabetes Study
VALIANT	VALsartan In Acute Myocardial INfarction Trial
VALUE	Valsartan Antihypertensive Long-term Use Evaluation
VEGF	vascular endothelial growth factor
VHL	von Hippel–Lindau
WHO	World Health Organization
WMH	white matter hyperintensity

Part 1
Epidemiology, pathogenesis, and diagnosis

CHAPTER 1

Epidemiology of hypertension

Sunil K. Nadar and Stephanie L. Harrison

KEY POINTS

* The prevalence of hypertension globally is high and increasing, particularly in low- and middle-income countries.
* Hypertension is a leading risk factor for cardiovascular disease and death worldwide.
* Hypertension is associated with a high risk of future cardiovascular events, and many modifiable and non-modifiable factors influence the development of hypertension.
* From a public health point of view, screening and patient education are important in the diagnosis, management, and prevention of hypertension.

1.1 Introduction

The global prevalence of hypertension was estimated to be 1.13 billion in 2015, with the overall prevalence of around 26% of the world's population and around 30–34% of those aged 18 years and above. Hypertension is a risk factor for many cardiovascular, cerebrovascular, and cardiovascular-related conditions, and substantially contributes to premature mortality. In 2017, it was estimated that hypertension is the leading modifiable risk factor for all-cause mortality world-wide, accounting for over 10 million deaths and 218 million disability-adjusted life years. It is believed that there is a global epidemic of yet unknown proportions as abnormally elevated blood pressures are often asymptomatic. Indeed, the first diagnosis of hypertension is often made when the individual presents with a myocardial infarction or a stroke. Hypertension is thus rightly often referred to as the 'silent killer'. Modifiable factors impacting hypertension include lifestyle changes such as smoking, diet, and physical activity levels. Public health initiatives for hypertension, such as population and opportunistic screening and patient education to promote 'heart-healthy' lifestyles, are critical for primary prevention, detection, and management of hypertension.

1.2 Historical perspective

The theories regarding blood circulation and blood pressure go far back in history. In ancient Greece, Hippocrates and Galen knew about arteries and veins. Galen was convinced veins and arteries were not connected and blood flowed both backward and forward from the heart. His teachings were unchallenged for more than 1000 years.

It was only during the Middle Ages that these teachings were challenged, and new experiments were conducted and these laid the basis for our modern understanding of the heart and circulation. It was William Harvey in 1616 who first described a one-way circulation of blood and correctly suggested the existence of capillaries. In 1733, Stephen Hales, an English clergyman, was the first person to measure blood pressure, albeit in a horse. Almost 150 years later, Ritter von Basch invented a machine that could measure the blood pressure of a human being in a non-invasive manner. This was the forerunner of the device introduced by Riva-Rocci in 1896, which proved to be a prototype of today's refined instruments. This, along with the invention of the stethoscope by René Laennec, helped Russian scientist N. S. Korotkoff in 1905 to monitor the pulse whilst the blood pressure cuff was inflated, giving birth to the term 'Korotkoff sounds'.

Before long, patients were having their blood pressure checked, and high blood pressure came to be known as 'hypertension'. At that time, it was felt that in certain conditions, raised blood pressure helped to maintain the perfusion of various organs and was not particularly harmful, hence the term 'benign essential hypertension', as opposed to 'malignant hypertension', which was thought to be very high blood pressures that could result in brain haemorrhage and heart failure.

It was only towards the middle of the twentieth century that various surgical and pharmacological interventions were considered for the treatment of hypertension, although its exact risk was uncertain. Some of the initial surgical procedures that were considered included thoracic sympathectomy, while drug therapy consisted mainly of sedatives. Diuretics were introduced for hypertension in the 1950s and 1960s, but scepticism still persisted in the medical community about the benefit of treating this 'benign essential' condition.

1.3 Hypertension and cardiovascular risk

It was not until the late 1970s and 1980s that large-scale epidemiological studies, including the Framingham study, clearly demonstrated the association between high blood pressure and cardiovascular risk. At the same time, a Veterans Administration study demonstrated that treating hypertensive patients with diuretics appeared to protect them from future events. These studies, and especially the more recent prospective studies collaboration by Lewington et al., have demonstrated that there is an almost linear relationship between blood pressure and cardiovascular and cerebrovascular risk. From the ages of 40–69, there is a twofold increase in mortality rates from ischaemic heart disease, and more than a twofold increase in stroke mortality for each 20 mmHg increase in systolic blood pressure and 10 mmHg increase in diastolic blood pressure. They also found that there is no evidence of a threshold wherein blood pressure is not directly related to risk, even at levels as low as 115/75 mmHg. They also concluded that a 10 mmHg higher systolic or 5 mmHg higher diastolic blood pressure would be associated, in the long term, with a higher risk of about 30% of death from ischaemic heart disease.

It is well established that hypertension is associated with a higher incidence of cardiovascular events, including myocardial infarction, heart failure and peripheral artery disease, cerebrovascular events, including haemorrhagic or ischaemic stroke, and cardiovascular-related conditions, including end-stage renal disease. Many of these associations have been demonstrated across multiple age and ethnic groups. Emerging evidence has also associated hypertension with an increased risk of atrial fibrillation, cognitive decline, and dementia.

It has also been shown that in people with low blood pressure who are not receiving any antihypertensive therapy, the incidence of cardiovascular disease is less. However, this cannot be used to support the benefits of therapy, as naturally occurring low blood pressure may offer a degree of protection that is not provided by a similarly low blood pressure resulting from antihypertensive therapy. However, many randomized controlled trials have demonstrated a significant benefit for treating individuals with high blood pressure, especially when they are at high risk of future cardiovascular events due to coexisting factors.

For an individual patient, the greatest risk is from a higher level of blood pressure. However, for the population at large, the greatest burden from hypertension occurs among people with only minimally elevated blood pressure, as they are more likely to develop overt hypertension in the following years and often the majority of them are picked up once they have had an event.

1.4 Prevalence of hypertension

The exact prevalence of hypertension is not clear, but the number of people with hypertension was estimated to be 1.13 billion in 2015, with the overall prevalence in adults of between 30% and 45%, with marked differences between countries. The prevalence of hypertension increases with age, and has been estimated at over 60% among adults aged 60 years and over. Epidemiological studies appear to suggest that the prevalence and absolute numbers of people with hypertension are increasing. In 2005, Kearney and colleagues estimated the number of people with hypertension by 2025 would be nearly 1.5 billion. Reasons for increases in the prevalence of hypertension include increasing age of the population, lifestyle exposures, including more sedentary lifestyles and higher sodium intake, and improved screening and detection of hypertension.

There are disparities in the prevalence of hypertension worldwide. The prevalence of people with hypertension is increasing in low- and middle-income countries and decreasing in high-income countries. Between 2000 and 2010, the age-standardized prevalence of hypertension decreased by 2.6% in high-income countries but increased by 7.7% in low- and middle-income countries. Substantial differences in awareness, treatment, and control of hypertension have been suggested to contribute to the disparities in changing prevalence of hypertension between high-income countries and low- and middle-income countries.

1.5 Risk factors for hypertension and risk reduction strategies

Multiple factors contribute to hypertension, including genetic and environmental factors. An estimated 35–50% of hypertension is inherited. Genome-wide association analysis have identified 118 genetic loci associated with blood pressure; however, this only explains approximately 3.6% of trait variance for blood pressure. Several genetic polymorphisms which might affect the synthesis of proteins such as angiotensinogen glucocorticoid receptors and kallikrein have been reported. Although identification of genetic loci offers potential new therapeutic targets and the possibility of precision medicine to modify the risk of hypertension, currently genetic testing for hypertension has no role in routine clinical care for patients.

Ethnic differences are seen in the prevalence of hypertension among different ethnic groups within the same community. In the United States, Native American Indians have the same or a slightly higher prevalence, compared to the general population, whilst Hispanics have the same or a slightly lower prevalence, compared to the general population. African Americans have among the highest prevalence of hypertension in the world.

Geographical variations have been reported in the prevalence of hypertension within the same ethnic group. For example, in the United Kingdom, prevalence rates are higher in Scotland and Northern England, as compared to the rest of the country. Dietary differences and other lifestyle differences, such as alcohol consumption and sedentary behaviours, may account for this difference. Age and sex are the other determinants, with blood pressure increasing with age. Men are also more likely to have higher blood pressure than women during their middle age. Above the age of 60 (after menopause), women and men have similar blood pressure and thereafter (above the age of 70 and 80), women tend to have higher blood pressure.

Lifestyle factors, including diet, physical activity, and alcohol consumption, contribute substantially to the risk of hypertension. Figure 1.1 provides an overview of modifiable and non-modifiable risk factors for hypertension and recommended lifestyle modifications to reduce the risk of hypertension. Lifestyle modifications to promote a 'heart-healthy' lifestyle can delay or prevent hypertension and subsequently reduce the risk of cardiovascular and cardiovascular-related diseases and events. The following lifestyle modifications are recommended in clinical guidelines to delay or prevent hypertension: (1) dietary modifications, including salt restriction and high consumption of fruits and vegetables; (2) reduced/moderated alcohol consumption; (3) maintaining optimal body weight; and (4) regular physical activity. Smoking may also raise blood pressure, and smoking and the

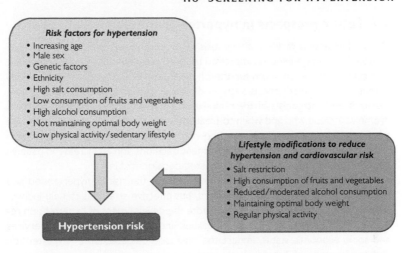

Figure 1.1 Non-modifiable and modifiable risk factors of hypertension and lifestyle strategies to reduce risk.

listed lifestyle modifications are recommended for prevention of other conditions beyond hypertension, including risk reduction for cardiovascular disease, cancer, and dementia.

1.6 Screening for hypertension

From a public health point of view, extensive screening and health education programmes on the importance of healthy lifestyle modifications should be considered for early detection of hypertension and primary prevention, respectively. Population screening, including mass screening and targeted screening, and opportunistic measurement of blood pressure are all possible screening approaches.

In a hypertension screening study of over 140,000 people, over 46% of people identified with hypertension were previously unaware of the diagnosis, and this was irrespective of whether the country was high-, middle-, or low-income. However, a review published in 2020 concluded that there is no high-certainty evidence to indicate whether mass, targeted, or opportunistic hypertension screening strategies are effective for reducing morbidity and mortality associated with hypertension. The 2018 European Society of Cardiology/European Society of Hypertension guidelines for hypertension recommend that all adults should have their blood pressure recorded at least every 5 years if they have an optimal blood pressure of <120/80 mmHg, or more frequently when opportunities arise. For adults with a blood pressure of 120–129/80–84 mmHg, measurement should be repeated every 3 years, and for adults with high-normal blood pressure of 130–139/85–89 mmHg, measurement should be repeated annually.

1.7 Future prospects in hypertension research

Our understanding of the pathogenesis of hypertension and its subsequent detection and management has improved tremendously over the past few decades. The current armamentarium for the physician in treating hypertension includes a wide array of medications such as diuretics, calcium channel blockers, beta blockers, and antagonists of the renin–angiotensin–aldosterone system. Current dilemmas include who and when to treat and with which medication(s) to initiate treatment, along with difficulties in knowing what targets to reach. Updated clinical guidelines help with directing treatment decisions and an increase in patient-centred care worldwide encourages shared decision-making.

Knowledge of lifestyle modifications to reduce the risk of hypertension and cardiovascular events is well established, but effective strategies to help individuals implement the lifestyle changes before the development of hypertension requires further research. Health inequalities, including access to health services and socio-economic status, impact the likelihood of detection of hypertension and the capacity of individuals to implement recommended lifestyle changes. Awareness, treatment, and control of hypertension has increased worldwide, but there are large disparities between high-income and low- and middle-income countries which should be addressed.

KEY REFERENCES

Beaney T, Schutte AE, Stergiou GS, et al. (2020). May Measurement Month 2019: The Global Blood Pressure Screening Campaign of the International Society of Hypertension. Hypertension 76:333–41.

Chow CK, Teo KK, Rangarajan S, et al.; PURE (Prospective Urban Rural Epidemiology) Study investigators (2013). Prevalence, awareness, treatment, and control of hypertension in rural and urban communities in high-, middle-, and low-income countries. JAMA 310:959–68.

Kannel WB (1996). Blood pressure as a cardiovascular risk factor: prevention and treatment. JAMA 275:1571–6.

Kearney PM, Whelton M, Reynolds K, et al. (2005). Global burden of hypertension: analysis of worldwide data. Lancet 365:217–23.

Lewington S, Clarke R, Qizihash N, et al. (2002). Age specific relevance of usual blood pressure to vascular mortality: a meta-analysis of individual data for one million adults in 61 prospective studies. Lancet 360:1903–13.

Mills KT, Bundy JD, Kelly TN, et al. (2016). Global disparities of hypertension prevalence and control: a systematic analysis of population-based studies from 90 countries. Circulation 134:441–50.

Schmidt B-M, Durao S, Toews I, et al. (2020). Screening strategies for hypertension. Cochrane Database Syst Rev 5:CD013212.

Stanaway JD, Afshin A, Gakidou E, et al. (2018). Global, regional, and national comparative risk assessment of 84 behavioural, environmental and occupational, and metabolic risks or clusters of risks for 195 countries and territories, 1990–2017: a systematic analysis for the Global Burden of Disease Study 2017. *Lancet* **392**:1923–94.

Vasan RS, Larson MG, Leip EP, *et al*. (2001). Assessment of frequency of progression to hypertension in non-hypertensive subjects in the Framingham Heart Study. A cohort study. *Lancet* **358**:1682–6.

Williams B, Mancia G, Spiering W, *et al*. (2018). 2018 ESC/ESH Guidelines for the management of arterial hypertension: The Task Force for the management of arterial hypertension of the European Society of Cardiology (ESC) and the European Society of Hypertension (ESH). *Eur Heart J* **39**:3021–104.

CHAPTER 2

Pathophysiology of hypertension

Sheon Mary, Giacomo Rossitto, and Christian Delles

KEY POINTS

- Blood volume, blood flow, and vascular resistance are tightly interlinked and together determine blood pressure.
- In most patients with hypertension, systems in the kidneys and the vasculature are dysregulated; blood pressure is raised by multiple factors, including salt/volume retention, vasoconstriction, and changes in cardiac output.
- In patients with primary hypertension, several subtle pathophysiological mechanisms come together, necessitating combination therapy to address different aspects of the pathophysiology.
- In patients with secondary hypertension, there is predominance of a single factor that drive the blood pressure increase; specifically addressing these factors can control their hypertension.

2.1 Introduction

Hypertension is defined as blood pressure above a certain prespecified threshold. In order to understand the pathophysiology of hypertension, it is therefore important to understand the physiology of blood pressure regulation. The latter is based on a complex network of regulatory elements, as illustrated in a model of circulatory control first proposed by Arthur Guyton and colleagues. In pragmatic contrast, we will employ a reductionist approach for the purpose of this chapter, in order to highlight a few key principles of blood pressure regulation that will help us to integrate current knowledge, be open for discoveries, and build a bridge between somewhat artificial concepts such as primary and secondary forms of hypertension.

2.2 A reductionist approach to the circulatory system

The mammalian cardiovascular system includes the pulmonary and systemic circulations which are connected by the heart. In clinical practice, we often see these as independent circulations, with respiratory physicians taking care of the former and cardiovascular physicians of the latter. From a physiological perspective, this separation is not correct as the two systems influence each other. However, for the purposes of this chapter, we will focus on the

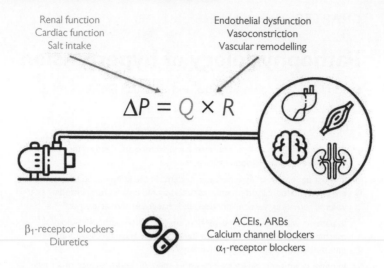

Renal function
Cardiac function
Salt intake

Endothelial dysfunction
Vasoconstriction
Vascular remodelling

$$\Delta P = Q \times R$$

β_1-receptor blockers
Diuretics

ACEIs, ARBs
Calcium channel blockers
α_1-receptor blockers

Figure 2.1 A reductionist approach to blood pressure regulation. If a fluid (blood) is supplied to the periphery through the driving force of a pump (heart), the flow (Q) is determined by the pressure gradient (ΔP) divided by the resistance of the tube (blood vessels) (R). As such, blood pressure is the product of flow and resistance, as illustrated in the figure. Three examples are given for factors that influence either part of the equation and thereby contribute to blood pressure control in normal physiology and hypertension in pathophysiological situations. The bottom part of the figure illustrates the key actions of antihypertensive agents on flow and resistance.

ACEI, angiotensin-converting enzyme inhibitor; ARB, angiotensin receptor blocker.

Icons made by Freepik and Vitaly Gorbachev from www.flaticon.com.

systemic circulation. A radically simple model, as discussed by Laragh, would therefore reduce the circulation to a system where a pump (heart) supplies a fluid (blood) via a tube (blood vessels) to the periphery (organs and tissues). In this model, flow (Q) is determined by the difference in pressure across the system (ΔP) divided by resistance (R). Pressure is the product of flow and resistance (Figure 2.1).

This reductionist model clearly indicates that any changes in pressure can only be the result of changes in flow or resistance, and we will use it in this sense to explore the pathophysiology of hypertension. There are, however, major conceptual flaws with this approach that we should bear in mind:

- The model is linear, and not a model of circulating blood. As mentioned earlier, it also does not take the connection to the pulmonary circulation into account.

- The model focusses on the arterial system (delivery to tissues) but disregards the important role of the venous and lymphatic systems within the circulation.

- The model replaces a complex system of branching arteries by a single tube between pump and periphery, and therefore disregards phenomena such as wave reflection at branching points.

- The model further assumes a continuous reduction of pressure along the tube, depending on its resistance, whereas the cardiovascular system is composed of high-flow/low-resistance vessels (e.g. large vessels such as the aorta or femoral arteries) and low-flow/high-resistance vessels (e.g. small vessels with a diameter <200 μm), with the majority of pressure reduction occurring in the latter.

- The model also does not account for organ-specific regulation of blood supply and the effect of local changes (e.g. carotid artery stenosis, coarctation of the aorta) on pressure and flow in other parts of the circulation.

The basic principle that pressure is determined by flow and resistance still holds true and we will comment on the above limitations as we discuss individual pathophysiological principles.

2.3 Flow and blood pressure

In our reductionist model, 'flow' is indeed dependent on two factors: volume and throughput (output) of the pump. Translating this to the cardiovascular system, both blood volume and cardiac output will have an effect on blood pressure. The effect of volume on blood pressure is well known in clinical practice: patients who suffer from acute blood loss have low blood pressure (haemorrhagic shock). Vice versa, an intravenous infusion of fluids increases blood pressure and is often one of the first measures to stabilize patients with severe hypotension.

If we consider less extreme situations and look at normal physiology, cardiac output indeed affects blood pressure. Seminal experiments demonstrated the acute effect of changes in heart rate or cardiac contractility on blood pressure and this plays an important role in short-term adaptation to higher demand. A key regulator of cardiac output is the sympathetic nervous system which regulates all major components of cardiac performance, including chronotropic (i.e. heart rate) and inotropic (i.e. contractility) responses. Release of adrenaline and noradrenaline in 'stress' situations can thereby increase blood pressure via a cardiac mechanism. This mechanism also explains, in part, why beta adrenergic receptor blockers lower blood pressure.

In the longer term, however, the 'flow' part of our model is mainly determined by volume, rather than by cardiac output, and volume regulation by the kidneys plays a more important role in maintaining a certain blood pressure level. The kidneys can effectively control sodium, and thereby volume, through the principle of pressure natriuresis whereby renal sodium (and, for osmosis, water) excretion is increased with increasing pressure to the kidney. In patients with acute or chronic kidney disease, this renal mechanism of volume control can be impaired and lead to salt- and volume-driven rise in blood pressure. Diuretics (which are largely natriuretics) therefore play an important role in lowering blood pressure.

At this point, it is important to mention that increased salt intake can affect blood pressure. In the vast majority of people, modest amounts of salt will not cause hypertension as the kidneys can increase sodium excretion and thereby prevent the volume effect of salt. However, some individuals are particularly salt-sensitive, with impaired pressure natriuresis; reduction in salt intake can contribute significantly to controlling their hypertension. As it is not practical to test every person for salt sensitivity, population-based strategies to reduce salt intake are a pragmatic way to reduce blood pressure—with smaller effects in most, but larger effects in salt-sensitive people. Whilst recently suggested tissue accumulation of sodium may have direct biological implications in the function of inflammatory/immune cells and/or vascular function beyond its simple intravascular volume effect, these aspects are still under investigation. From a pragmatic point of view, many of the effects of salt on blood pressure can still be explained by its more 'traditional' and kidney-centric effects. Indeed, many of the monogenic (Mendelian) disorders of blood pressure regulation are due to mutations in genes encoding sodium transporters in the kidney.

2.4 Vascular resistance and blood pressure

With pressure being determined by flow and resistance, any increase in vascular resistance will lead to an increase in blood pressure. This is certainly true in our reductionist model, but more complex in the cardiovascular system where multiple organs and tissues are perfused in parallel. It should also be noted that the three parameters flow, pressure, and resistance influence one another in order to preserve perfusion.

Vasoconstriction or vasodilation are effective means to increase or decrease blood pressure, respectively. Blood vessels are under the control of both local and systemic factors that regulate their tone. Locally, the endothelium produces vasoconstrictors, such as endothelin, and vasodilators such as nitric oxide. Systemically, the renin–angiotensin–aldosterone system (RAAS), with its principal effector angiotensin II, and the sympathetic nervous system via α_1 adrenergic receptors on smooth muscle cells are potent vasoconstrictors. Blockers of the RAAS and α_1 adrenergic receptor blockers are therefore used in the treatment of hypertension to counteract increased vasoconstriction, and vasodilators such as calcium channel blockers are another important class of antihypertensive agents acting directly at the level of the vasculature.

Whilst vasoconstriction and vasodilation are functional phenomena that are reversible, vascular remodelling and rarefication can have an irreversible effect on vascular resistance. Both can be the result of vessels being exposed to high pressure over prolonged periods of time where remodelling of small vessels and stiffening of large vessels can be observed as a consequence of hypertension. In a vicious circle, structurally increased vascular resistance then contributes itself to maintaining high blood pressure.

One ought to remember that seeing resistance and flow in isolation is helpful to understand the principles of blood pressure regulation, but all three factors of the equation are, of course, interconnected. The sympathetic nervous system and the RAAS are prime examples for these links. They will be activated in situations where higher blood pressure and higher organ perfusion are required, for example, in a 'fight or flight' situation with increased oxygen demand by the musculature. Activation of the sympathetic nervous system will increase not only cardiac output, but also vascular resistance, and in concert both factors will result in increased pressure and, if the balance is right, increase organ perfusion. In pathological situations, such as in patients with phaeochromocytoma, overproduction of adrenaline and noradrenaline disrupts this balance. Similarly, angiotensin II increases vascular resistance by vasoconstriction but also, via aldosterone, leads to sodium retention and increased volume, thereby again increasing blood pressure via both volume and resistance-based mechanisms. Again, in pathological situations with overproduction of angiotensin II, such as in patients with renal artery stenosis, complex situations with vasoconstriction and volume overload (including flash pulmonary oedema) can develop. In clinical practice, the interplay between volume and resistance explains why often combination therapies that address more than one primary mechanism are required to successfully treat patients with hypertension.

2.5 Key role of the vasculature in the pathogenesis of hypertension

The vasculature in its entirety contributes to blood pressure control and, in pathological situations, to hypertension and hypertensive organ damage in more complex ways beyond its direct role on vascular resistance. Small low-flow/high-resistance vessels, as alluded earlier, are the actual site of dynamic regulation of this resistance; microvascular function and structure are therefore of immediate relevance to the pathogenesis of hypertension.

Large vessels play no major role in such haemodynamic regulation. However, they are key in the propagation of pressure waves from the heart to the periphery. These pressure waves are reflected at points where resistance changes, namely at branching points where larger vessels divide into small-resistance arteries. The reflected pressure wave would normally return to the heart in diastole and provide pressure for perfusion of the coronary arteries. If large vessels are stiffer (e.g. as a result of chronic exposure to high blood pressure leading to fibrosis, in atherosclerosis, or because of calcification), pulse wave velocity will be increased and the reflected wave will reach the heart already during systole and thereby further increase systolic pressure (i.e. myocardial afterload). Modulating large artery stiffness is a promising theoretical concept to reduce blood pressure, but currently there are no drugs available that exclusively 'de-stiffen' blood vessels. However, some antihypertensive agents, such as RAAS blockers, exhibit antifibrotic actions, in addition to their blood pressure-lowering effects.

2.6 The kidney and hypertension

The kidneys are the main regulators of fluid and electrolyte homeostasis and, as such, directly affect blood pressure via intravascular and total body volume. There are multiple ways in how the normal regulatory role of the kidneys can be compromised and thereby lead to hypertension.

Electrolyte transport, and particularly the ability to excrete sodium, can be affected by rare mutations in electrolyte transporters in the renal tubule, for example, in Liddle syndrome where a gain-of-function mutation of the epithelial sodium channel leads to increased sodium reabsorption. The kidneys are, however, also involved in blood pressure control via the RAAS where any underperfusion (e.g. in renal artery stenosis) or loss of function (e.g. in chronic kidney disease or following subtotal nephrectomy) stimulates the release of renin, and thereby activation of the RAAS. These renal forms of hypertension can be particularly complex, as they are characterized by volume excess, sodium excess, vasoconstriction, and vascular stiffening, and therefore difficult to treat. Renal clearance of some antihypertensive agents and their effects (e.g. on the RAAS) can limit the number of antihypertensive drugs that can be used in these patients.

As we refer to hypertension as 'arterial hypertension', it appears counter-intuitive to discuss the role of the venous and lymphatic systems in this context. In fact, there is very little research into this part of the circulation that does more than just closing the loop and transporting blood back to the heart. Recent discoveries of a critical role of the lymphatic system in inflammation and sodium balance and its role in overall fluid balance are only the first steps towards a better understanding of the second part of our circulatory system.

2.7 Primary and secondary forms of hypertension

Most patients with hypertension have high blood pressure because of a combination of reasons. Many of these will be genetically determined, as evidenced by the high heritability of hypertension. Variants of multiple genes that encode proteins that are involved in blood pressure regulation can be found in the majority of patients with hypertension. Hypertension can, however, also develop from a combination of environmental causes such as increased salt intake, obesity, lack of exercise, and insulin resistance, especially when combined with a genetic predisposition. These patients with no single causative factor for their high blood pressure are thought to have 'primary hypertension' and treatment strategies focus on lifestyle modification and antihypertensive medication.

A much smaller percentage of patients with high blood pressure have 'secondary hypertension'. These will have one major driver of their high blood pressure but can still have other factors that contribute to it or have counterregulatory pathways activated as well. It is important to note that all forms of secondary hypertension can only act via the mechanisms described earlier. Key examples of secondary forms of hypertension include renal diseases, and particularly renal artery stenosis (via activation of the RAAS—vasoconstriction and sodium retention), primary aldosteronism (the archetype of a sodium-retaining condition), phaeochromocytoma (via increased cardiac output and vasoconstriction), and Cushing's syndrome (mainly via sodium and water retention). In addition, monogenic forms of hypertension mainly affecting renal electrolyte transport have been characterized.

In patients with secondary forms of hypertension, treatment of the underlying principal pathology can completely normalize blood pressure, and screening for such conditions is therefore important in clinical practice. However, from a pathophysiological perspective, the mechanisms involved in primary and secondary hypertension are similar—it is only the weighting of individual factors that is different.

2.8 New insights into the pathophysiology of hypertension

Research into the origins of hypertension has seen some change in focus over the last few decades. Initial focus on the sympathetic nervous system has moved to other pathophysiological concepts, including renal mechanisms and, more recently, the RAAS. Interestingly, at least in the initial genome-wide association studies (GWAS) into hypertension, none of these systems featured prominently and genes that were found to be associated with hypertension appeared to be involved in other, hitherto unrecognized, pathways, especially in signalling cascades. We have since learnt that the genetic factors underlying hypertension act much more indirectly on the principles discussed in the above sections, for example, by affecting intracellular signalling, rather than by simply being a missense mutation of the genes encoding renin, angiotensinogen, or adrenergic receptors. There are currently >1000 genetic loci firmly associated with hypertension or blood pressure, and much more work is needed to understand the molecular pathways linking these genes with the phenotype.

Mechanistic research in preclinical models provides deep insight into the pathogenesis of hypertension. For example, increased levels of reactive oxygen species, such as superoxide anion, interact with endothelium-derived nitric oxide and thereby reduce nitric oxide bioavailability, resulting in relative vasoconstriction. Inflammation (e.g. triggered by chronic exposure to microbial pathogens or as part of the atherosclerosis process) also affects endothelial function and can cause structural vascular changes (fibrosis). There is growing insight on how inflammation links diet and lifestyle (via the gut microbiome) and salt to hypertension.

We are also beginning to understand that hypertension is not just a risk factor for other cardiovascular diseases, but also often an integral element of such conditions. For example, the role of hypertension in the development of heart failure, and especially of heart failure with preserved ejection fraction, cannot be underestimated. There are also lessons to be learnt from hypertensive disorders of pregnancy, including pre-eclampsia—even if blood pressure seems to return to normal after delivery, affected women are at higher risk of developing hypertension later in life. Alterations in the balance between pro- and antiangiogenic factors, together with traditional risk factors for both pre-eclampsia and cardiovascular diseases, seem to explain this relationship.

Finally, new discoveries and findings from GWAS have sparked our interest again in mechanisms of hypertension that seemed forgotten for a while. GWAS into hypertension and chronic kidney disease have found an association between the gene encoding uromodulin and both conditions; research into the role of this abundant urinary protein in sodium homeostasis and other renal mechanisms of hypertension has led to new insights. The development of catheter-based renal denervation techniques offers new insights into the role of the sympathetic nervous system in the pathophysiology of hypertension. It also appears that the RAAS has further important effects on cardiovascular health through more recently discovered components such as angiotensin-converting enzyme 2 (ACE2) and its products, including Ang1-7 and Ang1-9.

2.9 Conclusion

The pathophysiology of hypertension has been discussed here with a fresh approach that does not focus on primary and secondary hypertension and clinical conditions, but based on physiological principles. Our reductionist approach can help to understand these principles which, in a complex organism, are of course interconnected. As such, we would always expect several pathologies coming together in order to lead to increased blood pressure.

Blood pressure regulation is an important part of normal physiology. Here the three components flow, pressure, and resistance are modulated, with the main aim to adapt organ and tissue perfusion to any changes in requirement. It is important to recognize that the pathophysiological mechanisms that ultimately lead to hypertension might already be present (but counterbalanced by other factors) at a stage where blood pressure is still within the normal range. Much deeper phenotyping to recognize such early stages could be the basis for truly preventative strategies to avoid the development of clinically overt hypertension.

KEY REFERENCES

Delles C, McBride MW, Graham D, Padmanabhan S, Dominiczak AF (2010). Genetics of hypertension: from experimental animals to humans. *Biochim Biophys Acta* **1802**:1299–308.

Foss JD, Kirabo A, Harrison DG (2017). Do high-salt microenvironments drive hypertensive inflammation? *Am J Physiol Regul Integr Comp Physiol* **312**:R1–4.

Guyton AC (1981). The relationship of cardiac output and arterial pressure control. *Circulation* **64**:1079–88.

Intengan HD, Schiffrin EL (2000). Structure and mechanical properties of resistance arteries in hypertension: role of adhesion molecules and extracellular matrix determinants. *Hypertension* **36**:312–18.

Laragh J (2001). Laragh's lessons in pathophysiology and clinical pearls for treating hypertension. *Am J Hypertens* **14**:397–404.

Laurent S, Boutouyrie P (2015). The structural factor of hypertension: large and small artery alterations. *Circ Res* **116**:1007–21.

Mahfoud F, Schlaich M, Böhm M, Esler M, Lüscher TF (2018). Catheter-based renal denervation: the next chapter begins. *Eur Heart J* **39**:4144–9.

McKinney CA, Fattah C, Loughrey CM, Milligan G, Nicklin SA (2014). Angiotensin-(1-7) and angiotensin-(1-9): function in cardiac and vascular remodelling. *Clin Sci (Lond)* **126**:815–27.

Padmanabhan S, Graham L, Ferreri NR, Graham D, McBride M, Dominiczak AF (2014). Uromodulin, an emerging novel pathway for blood pressure regulation and hypertension. *Hypertension* **64**:918–23.

Titze J (2015). A different view on sodium balance. *Curr Opin Nephrol Hypertens* **24**:14–20.

Wilck N, Matus MG, Kearney SM, et al. (2017). Salt-responsive gut commensal modulates TH17 axis and disease. *Nature* **551**:585–9.

Williams B, Mancia G, Spiering W, et al.; Authors/Task Force Members (2018). 2018 ESC/ESH Guidelines for the management of arterial hypertension: The Task Force for the management of arterial hypertension of the European Society of Cardiology and the European Society of Hypertension: The Task Force for the management of arterial hypertension of the European Society of Cardiology and the European Society of Hypertension. *J Hypertens* **36**:1953–2041.

CHAPTER 3

Secondary hypertension

Gurbhej Singh and Gurpreet Singh Wander

KEY POINTS

* Secondary hypertension should be suspected in individuals with severe and resistant hypertension, especially when it occurs at a young age.
* Before evaluation, one should rule out white coat hypertension and evaluate adherence to medications and drug-induced hypertension (non-steroidal anti-inflammatory drugs, alcohol, and oral contraceptive pills).
* Often clues are present that suggest a particular secondary cause of hypertension.
* Biochemical investigations should precede imaging where endocrine causes are suspected.

3.1 Introduction

Most patients with hypertension do not have a defined cause and are categorized as having primary or essential hypertension. Patients with a defined and potentially reversible cause fall into secondary hypertension. The reported incidence of secondary hypertension ranges from 5% to 15%. There are certain clinical indicators which may suggest secondary hypertension. The causes for secondary hypertension show variation according to age and sex. A high index of suspicion should be exercised for younger patients (age <30 years) with hypertension that is resistant to treatment.

The aetiology of secondary hypertension may be broadly classified into renal (parenchymal and vascular), vascular, endocrine, neurological, hereditary, and other causes. The clinical clues to suspect secondary hypertension are given in Table 3.1.

3.2 Renal causes of hypertension

Hypertension is observed in approximately 60–80% of patients with chronic kidney disease (CKD). It could be due to renal parenchymal disease or renal vascular disease and both of these will be discussed separately.

3.2.1 Renal parenchymal diseases

Renal parenchymal disorders are the most common cause of secondary hypertension. The presence of proteinuria and haematuria and a history of renal

Table 3.1 Pathophysiology of clinical clues to suspect secondary hypertension

Condition	Clinical clues
Coarctation of the aorta	Significant difference in blood pressure between two arms (>20 mmHg), with upper limbs greater than lower limbs. Arterial bruit Radiofemoral delay Radio-radial delay
Phaeochromocytoma	Palpitations, headache, Cafe-au-lai spots Neurofibromatosis
Obstructive sleep apnoea	Daytime somnolence Obesity Snoring
Cushing's syndrome	Abdominal striae Central obesity Moon facies
Polycystic kidney disease	Palpable kidneys
Renovascular hypertension	Renal artery bruit

dysfunction are indicators of renal parenchymal disease. Hypertension is more severe in glomerular diseases than in interstitial diseases (chronic pyelonephritis). The pathogenesis, although only partially understood, consists of multiple mechanisms with activation of the renin–angiotensin system (RAS), sympathetic activation, salt and fluid retention, increased endothelin-1 levels, endothelial dysfunction, and oxidative stress. Increased sympathetic activity is seen due to decreased sensitivity of baroreceptors in the kidney, activation of chemoreceptors, and reduced renalase (a flavoprotein expressed in the heart and kidney that metabolizes catecholamines) activity.

The control of blood pressure in patients with CKD slows the progression of renal dysfunction. CKD is an independent risk factor for cardiovascular disease. Chronic glomerulonephritis, autosomal dominant polycystic kidney disease, diabetic nephropathy, and obstructive uropathy are causes of parenchymal renal disease.

3.2.2 Renal vascular diseases

Renovascular hypertension (RVH) is seen in 1–2% of patients with hypertension. Diseases affecting renal vasculature may range from renal artery stenosis (RAS) to small-vessel intrarenal vasculitis. RAS should be suspected in patients with abdominal bruit (present in 50% of patients with RAS), rapid worsening of renal function after initiation of an angiotensin-converting enzyme inhibitor (ACEI) or angiotensin receptor blocker (ARB), a difference in renal size on imaging, and resistant hypertension. Fibromuscular dysplasia (FMD) is seen more often in younger patients than in older patients where atherosclerotic RAS is more common. Takayasu's arteritis is the most common cause of RVH in young patients in some countries such as India. Other causes may include aortitis, aortic dissection, thromboembolism, external compression by a mass lesion, and congenital malformations.

Anatomical assessment may be achieved by renal artery ultrasound, computed tomography (CT) angiography scan, or magnetic resonance angiography. Atherosclerotic RAS occurs at the origin of the renal artery and FMD is seen in the middle to distal part.

Medical management is the mainstay of treatment and often multiple drugs have to be used. Bilateral RAS is a contraindication to renin–angiotensin system blockade due to a rapid rise in creatinine levels and reduced renal function associated with their use in this condition. Revascularization procedures, such as renal angioplasty with or without stenting, can be performed. However, the Angioplasty and Stent for Renal Artery Lesions (ASTRAL) trial (2009) and the Cardiovascular Outcomes in Renal Atherosclerotic Lesions (CORAL) trial (2014) showed no benefit for angioplasty and stenting in terms of long-term outcomes or blood pressure control, but a significant amount of harm in the stenting group. At present, revascularization is recommended when blood pressure is resistant to medical treatment or in the presence of complications such as flash pulmonary oedema or rapidly worsening renal functions.

3.3 Endocrine causes of hypertension

Endocrine causes of hypertension consist of hormone-induced conditions which are reversible with correction of the respective hormonal disturbance. These include disorders of the adrenal, thyroid, pituitary, and parathyroid glands, among others.

3.3.1 Primary aldosteronism

Primary aldosteronism is characterized by hypertension, hypokalaemia, and hypomagnesaemia. Its prevalence varies from 2% to 3% in patients with hypertension. It can occur secondary to an adenoma secreting aldosterone or due to idiopathic adrenal hyperplasia. Screening test for primary aldosteronism includes measurement of plasma aldosterone concentration and plasma renin activity (PRA). The ratio of plasma aldosterone concentration to PRA is a useful screening test. A ratio of ≥30:1, with plasma aldosterone levels of ≥550 pmol/L, has 90% sensitivity and specificity for an aldosterone-producing adenoma. All drugs affecting the renin–angiotensin system need to be withheld at least 2 weeks before the test. The mineralocorticoid receptor blocker spironolactone should be stopped 2 months before the test. Sodium loading and captopril suppression tests are performed to measure the aldosterone concentration after saline infusion and captopril, administration respectively.

Further, imaging to localize an aldosterone-producing adenoma may be done in the form of CT or nuclear magnetic resonance imaging (MRI). Adrenal vein and inferior vena cava sampling for cortisol and aldosterone levels may help in lateralization of the adenoma. Treatment consists of surgical removal of unilateral adenomas. Spironolactone or eplerenone is useful to prepare for surgery and correction of hypokalaemia, as preoperative administration prevents sudden haemodynamic and electrolyte changes during the perioperative period. Figure 3.1 summarizes the steps of investigation of a patient suspected of having hyperaldosteronism. Other conditions which may cause hypertension and hypokalaemia include congenital adrenocortical hyperplasia (17α- and 11β-hydroxylase deficiency) and deoxycorticosterone (DOC)-producing tumours.

3.3.2 Cushing's syndrome

Excessive secretion of cortisol leads to Cushing's disease or syndrome. When it is adrenocorticotrophic hormone (ACTH)-dependent, it is called Cushing's disease, and when ACTH-independent, it is labelled as Cushing's syndrome. ACTH-dependent Cushing's disease involves an ACTH-producing pituitary adenoma or an ectopic ACTH-producing tumour. Cushing's syndrome includes adrenal adenoma or hyperplasia causing excessive cortisol production. The mechanism of hypertension includes activation of the renin–angiotensin system, excessive vasoconstriction due to angiotensin II and catecholamines, and impaired vasodilatation due to reduction in activity of Nitrous oxide (NO), the kallikrein–kinin system, and prostacyclin.

Cushing's syndrome should be suspected in patients with osteoporosis, hypertension, central obesity, muscle weakness, purple striae, ecchymosis, and impaired glucose tolerance. overnight dexamethasone suppression test is helpful in diagnosis and has a sensitivity of 98–99%. Further evaluation is done to diagnose ACTH-dependent or independent Cushing's syndrome. This includes measurement of ACTH concentration in plasma and imaging the pituitary or adrenal gland by CT or MRI. Management is directed at identification and localization of the cause of excess cortisol and its surgical excision. Adrenal and ectopic ACTH-producing sources are often removed laparoscopically. Trans-sphenoidal hypophysectomy is performed to remove the causative mass in the pituitary gland. Medical management includes control of hypertension by blockade of the renin–angiotensin system.

3.3.3 Phaeochromocytoma

Phaeochromocytoma is a tumour of chromaffin cells in the adrenal medulla secreting excessive catecholamines. Ten per cent of phaeochromocytomas are bilateral, 10% are extra-adrenal, 10% are malignant, and 10% are familial (rule of 10%). Patients with phaeochromocytoma usually present with paroxysmal and pulsating headache, paleness, palpitations, and excessive

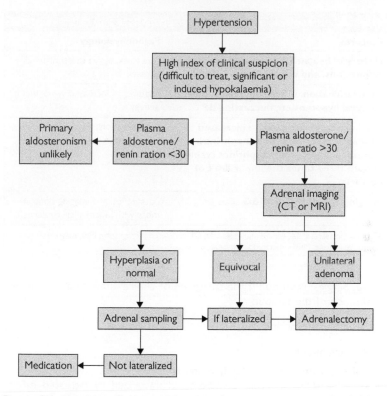

Figure 3.1 Algorithm for the diagnosis of a patient suspected of having hyperaldosteronism.

perspiration. It accounts for around 0.5–1% of patients with hypertension. It is sometimes seen as part of inherited disorders, including neurofibromatosis 1, von Hippel–Lindau (VHL) syndrome, and multiple endocrine neoplasia (MEN) type 2. Screening tests include measurement of metanephrines and normetanephrines in plasma and 24-hour urine. To confirm, the clonidine suppression test or chromogranin levels may be measured. CT or nuclear MRI can help localize the phaeochromocytoma. MIBG (^{123}I or ^{131}I-metaiodobenzylguanidine) scintigraphy and positron emission tomography (PET) of the adrenal glands (fluoro-dopamine PET) may further help localize the phaeochromocytoma (Table 3.2). Management includes initiation of alpha receptor antagonists (phentolamine) for 7–14 days to prevent the effect of excessive catecholamines on alpha receptors leading to a hypertensive crisis or cardiac arrhythmias. Subsequently, beta blockers may be

Table 3.2 Pathophysiology of steps in the diagnosis of phaeochromocytoma

Features	Pathophysiology
History of headache, sweating, anxiety, palpitations, and weight loss	Due to excessive catecholamine release
On examination: thin, tachycardia, pallor, postural hypotension, fluctuating BP	Features of increased sympathetic activity
Biochemical investigations: increased 24-hour urinary total metanephrines, increased plasma metanephrines (values of both three times the upper limit of normal)	Mild elevations are not diagnostic. Urinary VMA no longer used for diagnosis
Imaging: CT or MRI ± MIBG scan	Localization and imaging done in those with biochemical evidence

BP, blood pressure; VMA, vanillyl mandellic acid; CT, computed tomography; MRI, magnetic resonance imaging; MIBG, metaiodobenzylguanidine.

added. Surgical resection is the treatment of choice after identification and localization of the tumour.

3.3.4 Other endocrine causes

3.3.4.1 Acromegaly

Excessive growth hormone (GH) production from pituitary or GH-secreting tumours leads to this clinical syndrome, characterized by increased cardiac output, increased myocardial mass, and reduced peripheral vascular resistance. Hypertension is seen clinically in up to 40% of patients with acromegaly and these patients usually have diastolic dysfunction. Increased levels of GH and insulin-like growth factor 1 (IGF-1) are seen. Failure of suppression of GH after a glucose load should raise suspicion of a GH-producing tumour and imaging in the form of CT or MRI should be done to localize the site of production. Management includes medical therapy in the form of somatostatin analogues and GH receptor antagonists. Microsurgical trans-sphenoidal resection can be considered where medical therapy is not successful.

3.3.4.2 Diseases of the thyroid

Hyperthyroidism may cause systolic hypertension with a wide pulse pressure. Patients will have systemic features to suggest hyperthyroidism. Diagnosis is confirmed by measuring thyroid-stimulating hormone (TSH) levels, as well as free T3 and T4 levels. Management includes anti-thyroid drugs or surgery, depending on the cause of hyperthryoidism. Non-selective beta blockers may be used to control symptoms and hypertension, as they block peripheral conversion of T4 to T3 concurrently with anti-thyroid therapy.

Hypothyroidism may cause diastolic hypertension and is seen in around 30% of patients with hypothyroidism. Clinical features include malaise, cold intolerance, goitre, weight gain, hoarseness, constipation, and bradycardia. Diastolic hypertension occurs due to increased peripheral vascular resistance. There is reduced renin release and increased salt sensitivity. Management includes levothyroxine replacement and dose titration according to TSH levels.

3.3.4.3 Hyperparathyroidism

Parathyroid hormone (PTH) is known to have vasoconstrictor activity by affecting intracellular and serum calcium levels. Patients with primary hyperparathyroidism have higher PRA and noradrenaline levels, and hypertension has been reported in around 40–65% of these patients. Surgical removal of the parathyroid gland or adenoma is the mainstay of treatment. However, hypertension may persist, even after parathyroidectomy, in up to 50% of patients.

3.3.4.4 Renin-producing tumours

This tumour arises from the juxtaglomerular cells and is diagnosed by the presence of elevated aldosterone levels and PRA. Patients present with hypertension and hypokalaemia. Imaging helps to localize the tumour and management involves surgical removal of the tumour.

3.3.4.5 Carcinoid syndrome

Carcinoid syndrome occurs due to secretion of serotonin, bradykinin, and other neurohormones. It is a rare cause of secondary hypertension and clinically manifests as weight loss, flushing sensation, diarrhoea, bronchospasm, and features suggesting right heart failure. Surgery, chemotherapy, and blockers of serotonin are treatments for this condition.

3.4 Neurological causes of hypertension

The sympathetic nervous system controls blood pressure via baroreceptors and chemoreceptors. Baroreceptors are located in the media and adventitia of the internal carotid arteries (carotid sinus) and aortic arch, and are sensitive to distension of the vessel wall. They are stretch receptors on the terminal part of afferent fibres. In case of a fall in blood pressure, these afferent fibres fire less, leading to increased sympathetic activation as input of these afferent fibres cause reflex inhibition of the sympathetic system. Increase in intracranial pressure secondary to tumour, encephalitis, bleeding, or injury leads to activation of the sympathetic system, raising the systemic blood pressure. Conditions causing autonomic dysfunction such as familial dysautonomia, multiple system atrophy, primary autonomic failure or secondary to systemic diseases such as diabetes may cause hypertension. Spinal cord lesions involving cervical or upper thoracic levels may cause autonomic hyperreflexia, leading to high blood pressure levels.

3.5 Drug-induced hypertension

Many drugs and toxins can lead to hypertension. The mechanism of hypertension may be due to the effect of drugs on vascular tone (vasoconstriction or impaired vasodilatory properties of vessels), increase in sympathetic activity, effect on the circulating volume of blood, cardiac contractility, increase in red blood cell mass, reduction in parasympathetic activity, or retention of salt and water. Removing exposure to these agents in most cases will treat the hypertension, although occasionally hypertension is permanent. The different agents and the mode of causing hypertension are summarized in Table 3.3.

3.6 Hereditary causes of hypertension

Various hereditary causes for hypertension have been studied. In siblings with hypertension, genetic factors play a significant role. Monogenic hypertension has an identifiable genetic defect and causes hypertension by electrolyte alteration and water retention. It is further classified as low renin monogenic hypertension, with subclassification into low, normal, and high aldosterone level. The second type is monogenic hypertension with excessive sympathetic activity. Low renin with low aldosterone levels include Liddle's syndrome, congenital adrenal hyperplasia, Gellers syndrome, and apparent mineralocorticoid excess. Low renin with

Table 3.3 Drugs and external agents causing secondary hypertension	
Agent	Mechanism of causing hypertension
Glucocorticoids or mineralocorticoids	Salt and water retention Aldosterone receptor activation
Vitamin D	Increased cytosolic calcium, causing vasoconstriction
Levodopa, phenylephrine, selective serotonin reuptake inhibitors, bromocriptine, nicotine	Sympathetic system activation
Monoamine oxidase inhibitors	Prolonged half-life of noradrenaline
Anticholinergic drugs	Reduction in vasodilatory parasympathetic action
Calcineurin inhibitors	Fluid retention and vasoconstriction
Antacids containing sodium and bicarbonate	Fluid retention
Non-steroidal anti-inflammatory agents	Fluid retention and prostaglandin inhibition
Oral contraceptive pill	Salt and water retention
Heavy metals such as lead and mercury	Increased levels of adrenaline and noradrenaline

normal aldosterone levels is seen in Gordon's syndrome, and with high aldosterone levels in familial hyperaldosteronism types I, II, III, and IV. Management is directed according to alterations in each type of monogenic hypertension in the glucocorticoid, mineralocorticoid, and sympathetic pathways.

3.7 Diseases of the aorta causing hypertension

Structural changes in the vessel wall can lead to rigidity causing stiffness, thus preventing relaxation, and can increase blood pressure. This has been studied in patients with CKD, diabetes, and coronary artery disease. Changes in the arterial wall include alteration in the elastin:collagen ratio, increase in matrix collagen, smooth muscle hypertrophy, and changes in glycosaminoglycans. These changes may also occur with ageing due to arteriosclerosis. Measurement of pulse wave velocity non-invasively reflects large vessel stiffness.

Coarctation of the aorta is narrowing of the aorta anywhere along the course of the aorta; however, the most common site is near the left subclavian artery origin. It is the most common congenital cause of secondary hypertension. It is usually sporadic but occurs in 35% of those with Turner's syndrome. Its diagnosis is made clinically, with a difference in upper and lower limb blood pressures and auscultation of a systolic bruit over the front and back of the chest. It is usually diagnosed during early childhood clinically. All patients of coarctation of the aorta should be screened for bicuspid aortic valve disease. Echocardiography is a useful tool to screen for coarctation of the aorta, especially in infants and early childhood. Imaging of coarctation can be done by CT or MR aortic angiography. Clinically and haemodynamically significant coarctation of the aorta should be treated with balloon angioplasty/stenting or surgical repair.

3.8 Other causes of hypertension

Obstructive sleep apnoea (OSA) is a disease characterized by upper airway collapse during sleep, leading to apnoea and hypopnoea. More than 50% of patients diagnosed with OSA have hypertension. There is increased sympathetic activity seen in OSA, along with changes in the circadian pattern of blood pressure. Clinical presentation is with obesity, daytime somnolence, and hypertension. Seventy per cent of patients with OSA are obese. Diagnosis is made by the Epworth Sleepiness Scale (ESS) and polysomnography with the Apnoea-Hypopnoea Index (AHI). Early identification and management using weight reduction, lifestyle changes, and, if indicated, continuous positive airway pressure may help achieve blood pressure targets.

Certain high-output states may also cause hypertension, including beriberi disease due to thiamine deficiency, Paget's disease, and arteriovenous fistulae. In high-cardiac output states, there is an increase in cardiac output and a reduction in peripheral resistance, causing an increase in systolic blood pressure and a reduction in diastolic blood pressure.

3.9 Conclusion

Secondary hypertension involves complex mechanisms involving multiple systems, including endocrine, nervous, renal, respiratory, and vascular, acting together. Thus, identification of clinical features should guide relevant investigations. A secondary cause of hypertension should be suspected in young patients and where hypertension appears to be resistant to treatment. The goal in management of all cases of secondary hypertension remains control of blood pressure to target levels by a cost-effective management strategy and treatment of the underlying cause which, in many cases, can cure the hypertension.

KEY REFERENCES

Carey RM, Calhoun DA, Bakris GL, et al. (2018). Resistant hypertension: detection, evaluation, and management: a scientific statement from the American Heart Association. Hypertension 72:e53–90.

Funder JW, Carey RM, Mantero F, et al. (2016). The management of primary aldosteronism: case detection, diagnosis, and treatment: an Endocrine Society Clinical Practice Guideline. J Clin Endocrinol Metab 101:1889–916.

Rimoldi SF, Scherrer U, Messerli FH (2014). Secondary arterial hypertension: when, who, and how to screen? Eur Heart J 35:1245–54.

Shah SN, Munjal YP, Kamath SA, et al. (2019). Indian guidelines on hypertension-IV. J Hum Hypertens 34:745–58.

Viera AJ, Neutze DM (2010). Diagnosis of secondary hypertension: an age-based approach. Am Fam Physician 82:1471–8.

CHAPTER 4

Diagnosis and investigation of hypertension

Martin Wolley and Michael Stowasser

KEY POINTS

- The diagnosis of hypertension requires multiple readings.
- Out-of-office readings by ambulatory or home blood pressure monitoring are more representative of a patient's true blood pressure status than office readings and reduce the incidence of white coat hypertension.
- Investigations for hypertension should consider potential causes and evidence of end-organ damage, and assess for overall cardiovascular risk.

4.1 Introduction

Hypertension is the leading treatable risk factor for cardiovascular mortality worldwide. It is also one of the most frequently encountered medical conditions by physicians, and all clinicians treating adult patients should have expertise in the correct diagnosis and appropriate management of hypertension. As a continuous variable, blood pressure necessitates a cut-off value above which hypertension is diagnosed, and this has changed over time, with continued debate about a lower limit at which the diagnosis of hypertension should be conferred. Blood pressure also varies considerably, depending on the hour of the day and numerous other minor variables, and thus great care is required when interpreting blood pressure measurements.

4.2 Correct measurement of blood pressure

Accurate blood pressure measurement requires attention to detail to ensure that it is measured in a standardized and repeatable fashion. Important points on which to focus include:

- Use of a calibrated machine
- Appropriate cuff size (encircling 80% of the circumference of the arm and with the width at least 40% of the mid-upper arm circumference), especially in obese individuals where a sufficiently large cuff is required

- The patient relaxed and seated for at least 5 minutes, with their back resting against a chair
- No caffeine or smoking for 2 hours prior to testing
- At least two readings 5 minutes apart per measurement
- Measuring blood pressure in both arms when measuring the first time and taking the highest arm if the difference is >5 mmHg
- Considering measurement of seated and standing blood pressure (after 2 minutes' standing), especially in older patients

Blood pressure varies significantly over time in individuals, with a general circadian rhythm generally comprising a night-time dip and a morning surge, but also significant day-to-day variability driven by other factors such as activity level, anxiety, stress, exercise, etc. Because of this variability, a key component to the diagnosis of hypertension is the need for repeated blood pressure readings. Furthermore, blood pressure tends to be higher on the first visit to a clinician and to fall on repeated visits over time, with a median (interquartile range) drop of −8 mmHg (2–17 mmHg) in one recent study. For this reason, the diagnosis of hypertension based on office blood pressure readings requires repeated measurement over a reasonable time period. Generally, at least two sets of readings at least a week apart are needed before office hypertension can be confirmed, and most of the latest guidelines suggest confirming the diagnosis of hypertension with out-of-office readings. An exception may be made where blood pressure is substantially elevated in combination with clear evidence of end-organ damage, such as hypertensive retinopathy or acute renal dysfunction, which might necessitate more urgent treatment.

4.3 Criteria for diagnosis of hypertension

Hypertension has been defined by most guidelines based on office readings as a systolic above 140 mmHg or a diastolic above 90 mmHg (Table 4.1). In 2017, the American College of Cardiology and the American Heart Association categorized hypertension differently in their updated guideline, reflecting a push to more aggressive early lifestyle management, defining stage 1 hypertension as a systolic of 130–139 mmHg or a diastolic of 80–89 mmHg. This has been controversial and has not been followed by other major guidelines to date.

4.4 Alternatives and complements to office blood pressure measurement

Because of the natural variability of blood pressure, accuracy increases with the number of measurements over time. Ambulatory measurement with repeated readings over a 24-hour period or home blood pressure monitoring with repeated readings over a much longer period have significant advantages over office-based

Table 4.1 Conventional diagnostic categories for office blood pressure measurement according to the European Society of Hypertension/European Society of Cardiology guidelines 2018

Diagnostic category	Systolic (mmHg)		Diastolic (mmHg)
Normal	≤129	and	≤84
High-normal	130–139	and/or	85–89
Grade 1 (mild)	140–159	and/or	90–99
Grade 2 (moderate)	160–179	and/or	100–109
Grade 3 (severe)	≥180	and/or	≥110
Isolated systolic	>140	and	<90

Adapted with permission from Williams, B. Mancia G, Spiering W, et al. ESC Scientific Document Group, 2018 ESC/ESH Guidelines for the management of arterial hypertension: The Task Force for the management of arterial hypertension of the European Society of Cardiology (ESC) and the European Society of Hypertension (ESH), *European Heart Journal*, Volume 39, Issue 33, 01 September 2018, Pages 3021–3104, https://doi.org/10.1093/eurheartj/ehy339.

blood pressure measurement because of the larger number of readings and the ability to exclude white coat hypertension. Although white coat hypertension is defined as normal ambulatory blood pressure with high office readings, a 'white coat effect' is a frequent finding in all stages of hypertension, and thus out-of-office readings can help guide appropriate treatment. This is especially useful to diagnose true drug-resistant hypertension and to avoid overtreatment.

4.5 Ambulatory blood pressure measurement

Ambulatory blood pressure measurement (ABPM) is usually applied for a 24-hour period, and the machines are usually programmed to take readings every 30 minutes during the day, and often less frequently at night. Apart from the 24-hour average, useful information about the circadian pattern can be gained, with special importance to night-time blood pressure. An arbitrarily defined level of a >10% drop in average night-time pressures versus the daytime average is defined as a nocturnal dip, also called the 'dipping status', and absence of a nocturnal dip is associated with a significant increase in cardiovascular risk. Some studies further suggest that nocturnal blood pressure is more predictive than daytime or 24-hour average blood pressure, and thus night-time blood pressures might possibly be the most sensitive blood pressure measurement of all when considering cardiovascular risk.

Particular situations where ABPM is very useful include evaluation of hypertension where white coat hypertension is suspected, where there is apparent treatment-resistant hypertension, or where there is significant variation in office

Table 4.2 Criteria for hypertension based on ambulatory blood pressure measurement and home blood pressure monitoring

Method	Systolic (mmHg)		Diastolic (mmHg)
Office blood pressure	≥140	and/or	≥90
ABPM daytime	≥135	and/or	≥85
ABPM night-time	≥120	and/or	≥70
ABPM 24-hour average	≥130	and/or	≥80
Home blood pressure	≥135	and/or	≥85
ABPM, ambulatory blood pressure measurement.			

readings. ABPM may also be useful in so-called 'masked hypertension' where ambulatory pressures are high despite normal office readings. The prevalence of masked hypertension is unclear, but it appears to be more common in patients with diabetes and chronic kidney disease, and possibly in those with high-normal office blood pressures. Masked hypertension is associated with an increased risk of cardiovascular events, compared to normotension, but it is still a relatively understudied phenomenon.

The advantages of ABPM have led to the recommendation in many guidelines that a substantial proportion of hypertensives should be evaluated with ABPM, although widespread availability and relatively low cost of home blood pressure monitoring also offer an alternative or complementary method to ABPM. Correct use of ABPM does require some technical expertise and the device should be applied by an experienced nurse or technician, and the machines are much more expensive than home blood pressure monitors. Some patients also find the devices cause sleep disturbance, thus limiting the accuracy of night-time readings. Because ABPM readings tend to be lower than office readings, the diagnostic cut-offs for hypertension based on ABPM are also different (Table 4.2).

4.6 Home blood pressure measurement

Home blood pressure devices have become increasingly common and affordable, and provide a useful adjunct to office readings. A growing body of evidence demonstrates that home blood pressure measurement is more predictive of cardiovascular risk than standardized office readings and correlates more closely with end-organ damage. A validated upper arm device should be recommended to patients and, as with office readings, at least two readings taken 5 minutes apart after 5 minutes of rest are recommended for accuracy. Blood pressures can be measured at different times of the day, but a good general recommendation is first thing in the morning before medications and late in the day. Patients should record readings for review by their physician, with readings taken over at least 3 days and preferably over a week prior to a clinic visit, which is especially helpful in making treatment decisions. Newer and more advanced devices have the capability of linking with mobile phones or computers to provide aggregate data and calculate summary statistics. Some evidence also suggests that self-monitoring of blood pressure may be beneficial in terms of medication adherence and optimal blood pressure control, by providing a feedback loop directly to patients. Home blood pressure monitoring is also a highly valuable technique to facilitate telehealth appointments.

4.7 Automated office blood pressure measurement

The accuracy and reproducibility of office blood pressure measurement can be improved with use of automated devices recording multiple readings in a short sequence. If the patient is seated alone and unobserved, the white coat effect can also be reduced significantly. The optimal technique requires the patient to be seated quietly in a room by themselves for 5 minutes before several readings (typically three) are taken in sequence. The average of automated office blood pressure (AOBP) readings is similar to that obtained from daytime ambulatory readings or home blood pressure monitoring, and is substantially lower than those obtained by traditional office measurement. Exactly how much lower is not completely clear, but studies suggest it may be as much as 5–15 mmHg. Despite the difference between traditional office and AOBP readings, there is a sparsity of outcome data specifically for AOBP measurements, and thus specific cut-offs for diagnosis and treatment targets have not been formulated. Compared to ABPM, AOBP measurement is relatively inexpensive and simple to deploy in routine clinical settings.

4.8 Investigation of hypertension

Important clues to the aetiology of hypertension may be obtained from a careful history. Most patients with hypertension are asymptomatic, unless a severe and rapid increase in blood pressure occurs. Specific symptoms may give a clue to a hypertension aetiology. Nocturia is common in primary aldosteronism and chronic kidney disease, and patients with phaeochromocytoma classically (but not always) have a triad of headache, palpitations, and diaphoresis. Hypertension in a young woman may raise suspicion of an underlying fibromuscular disease of the renal arteries, whereas the presence of multiple cardiovascular risk factors and known vascular disease elsewhere in an older person may herald atherosclerotic renovascular disease.

A strong hereditary component to hypertension is well established, and a history of early cardiovascular disease, and especially haemorrhagic stroke, might point to an inherited high genetic risk of essential hypertension or rarer monogenetic forms such as glucocorticoid remedial aldosteronism. A full review of medications, including contraceptives, over-the-counter drugs, and supplements, should be undertaken. A dietary history to quantify the level of processed food

intake and estimate salt intake is useful, and enquiry into specific factors such as alcohol intake and liquorice ingestion is often fruitful. Sleep apnoea is common, and
symptoms easily elicitable. Several simple questionnaires, such as the Epworth
Sleepiness Scale and the STOP-BANG score, have good sensitivity for sleep apnoea and can be used easily in the clinic setting.

4.9 Clinical examination

Clinical examination in the initial assessment for hypertension should focus on the
search for findings suggesting end-organ damage or a possible secondary cause,
and also on assessing for other cardiovascular risk factors.

Weight, body mass index, and waist circumference are useful parameters to
record and can be monitored longitudinally, and also help in risk assessment
for obstructive sleep apnoea. Fundoscopic examination may reveal evidence
of hypertensive retinopathy. A detailed cardiovascular examination should be
undertaken, including examination of peripheral pulses and careful auscultation
for carotid, renal, and femoral bruits.

A unilateral reduced radial pulse and lower brachial blood pressure are usually from a subclavian stenosis and this may be accompanied by a subclavian
bruit. Aortic coarctations are more common in patients with Turner's syndrome.
Endocrine conditions such as Cushing's disease and acromegaly have classical
examination findings, and examining for thyrotoxicosis is also important.

4.10 Investigations

All patients with an established diagnosis of hypertension should have an assessment of renal function, including a urine sample. Acute and chronic kidney disease is almost invariably associated with hypertension and this can be the sole
presenting manifestation in some patients. A urine dipstick is a low-cost method
to exclude significant proteinuria and haematuria, although in diabetic patients,
a spot urine albumin:creatinine ratio should be performed due to its greater
sensitivity and specificity for albuminuria, and this should also be performed if a
urine dipstick is positive to more accurately quantify the degree of albuminuria.
Biochemistry should include a fasting glucose and lipid assessment, to adequately
assess the absolute cardiovascular risk in primary hypertension. An electrocardiogram (ECG) may be useful to look for evidence of left ventricular hypertrophy
(LVH), although other methods such as echocardiography are more sensitive,
albeit more expensive.

Further investigations depend on the clinical scenario and resources available.
Secondary hypertension is more common in patients with severe or resistant
hypertension, younger patients (<40 years) without other risk factors, and those
with electrolyte disorders, and in resource-limited settings, an extensive search
for secondary causes should be limited to patients in those categories. This is

Table 4.3 Suggested investigations for comprehensive assessment of hypertension and cardiovascular risk

Investigation	Purpose
Sodium, potassium, creatinine, eGFR	To exclude electrolyte disturbance and assess renal function
Fasting blood glucose ± HbA1c	To screen for diabetes
Lipids and subfractions	To assess cholesterol and cardiovascular risk
Urine analysis with microscopy and dipstick	To screen for haematuria and proteinuria
Urine albumin:creatinine ratio	More accurate quantification of albuminuria
24-hour urine collection for albumin, creatinine, sodium, and potassium	Most accurate measurement of albuminuria and electrolytes; objectively measures salt intake
12-lead ECG	To screen for LVH and other cardiac abnormalities
Echocardiography	To screen for LVH and valve disease
Renal artery Doppler study	To screen for renal artery disease and assess for other renal abnormalities where indicated
Aldosterone/renin ratio	To screen for primary aldosteronism
24 hour catecholamines and metanephrines	In resistant hypertension or where symptoms suggest phaeochromocytoma
1 mg overnight dexamethasone suppression test	In resistant hypertension or where symptoms or signs suggest Cushing's syndrome

eGFR, estimated glomerular filtration rate; ECG, electrocardiogram; LVH, left ventricular hypertrophy.

discussed in detail in Chapter 3. Table 4.3 lists some of the investigations that patients with newly diagnosed hypertension ought to have.

4.11 Assessing hypertension-mediated organ damage

It is important to assess newly diagnosed patients with hypertension for evidence of hypertension-mediated organ damage (HMOD). Evidence of HMOD in a newly diagnosed hypertensive patient can suggest that hypertension has been long-standing. Evaluation of HMOD is also useful as it helps to define the cardiovascular risk (see below) and can also predict prognosis. In some cases, regression of HMOD, such as LVH, is associated with improved prognosis. Suggested basic tests include ECG and echocardiography to assess for evidence of LVH and atrial fibrillation, carotid Doppler to assess for atheroma if clinically suspected, assessment of renal function (both blood and urine analysis and imaging), and retinoscopy. Some of the more advanced tests to assess for HMOD include measurement of the ankle–brachial index (to assess for peripheral vascular disease), cognitive function testing and brain imaging (to assess for cerebrovascular disease), and pulse-wave velocity measurement to assess for aortic stiffness. Although current guidelines do not recommend that these tests should be undertaken annually, it would be prudent for the basic work-up to be done on first diagnosis and further when clinically indicated.

4.12 Assessing cardiovascular risk

Assessing the absolute cardiovascular risk is an important task when a treatment plan for HMOD is not established. This is appropriate for patients with no known cardiovascular disease, chronic kidney disease, or other high-risk conditions. Excellent, easy-to-use risk calculators are available in many countries using country-specific data, and general calculators based on the Framingham risk cohort data are also available. Care does need to be taken to consider other risk factors not included in all calculators such as family history of early-onset cardiovascular disease or high-risk ethnic groups.

4.13 Conclusion

The diagnosis of hypertension requires measurement of blood pressure under strict conditions, and often multiple readings, including ambulatory 24-hour and home readings. Further investigations will be guided by the suspicion of secondary hypertension and in cases of resistant hypertension. Investigations to look for evidence of HMOD and to help calculate the cardiovascular risk are also indicated.

KEY REFERENCES

National Institute for Health and Care Excellence (2019). Hypertension in adults: diagnosis and management. NICE guideline [NG136]. Available from: https://www.nice.org.uk/guidance/ng136

Whelton PK, Carey RM, Aronow WS, et al. (2018). The 2017 ACC/AHA/AAPA/ABC/ACPM /AGS/APhA/ASH/ASPC/NMA/PCNA guideline for the prevention, detection, evaluation, and management of high blood pressure in adults: a report of the American College of Cardiology/American Heart Association Task Force on Clinical Practice Guidelines. *Hypertension* **71**:e13–115.

Williams B, Mancia G, Spiering W, et al.; ESC Scientific Document Group. (2018). 2018 ESC/ESH guidelines for the management of arterial hypertension. *Eur Heart J* **39**:3021–104.

Part 2
Complications of hypertension

Part 2

Complications of
Hepatectomy

CHAPTER 5

Hypertension: a cardiovascular risk factor

Thomas Salmon, James Hatherley, and Rajiv Sankaranarayan

KEY POINTS

* Hypertension is a major risk factor for cardiovascular disease.
* Both systolic and diastolic blood pressures impact cardiovascular risk.
* Hypertension typically occurs in the presence of other cardiovascular risk factors.
* Assessment tools, such as QRISK3 and SCORE, are useful in assessing cardiovascular risk.
* Appropriate management of hypertension leads to a reduction in cardiovascular risk.

5.1 Introduction

Hypertension is the leading risk factor for, and the most prevalent preventable cause of, cardiovascular disease worldwide. Cardiovascular disease accounts for a significant proportion of hypertension-related mortality, with the most common causes of premature death attributed to hypertension being ischaemic heart disease, ischaemic stroke, and haemorrhagic stroke. Hypertension is the premier risk factor in the development of heart failure (both with preserved (HFpEF) and reduced (HFrEF) ejection fraction), and a leading contributor to the development of ischaemic heart disease, cerebrovascular disease, and arrhythmia.

The Global Burden of Disease (GBD) 2019 study found that ischaemic heart disease and stroke are the second and third leading causes of disability-adjusted life years (DALYs) worldwide, respectively, behind neonatal disorders. Systolic hypertension is the leading risk factor contributing to worldwide morbidity, accounting for 9.3% of the global DALY burden. Over 75% of hypertension-associated DALYs are attributed to cardiovascular disease.

5.2 Hypertension and ischaemic heart disease

Ischaemic heart disease remains the highest single cause of systolic hypertension-related mortality worldwide. Much of the modern understanding of cardio-vascular risk factors is built on the findings of the Framingham Heart Study, an ongoing cardiovascular cohort study now spanning three generations, the first recruited in 1948. The Framingham study has shown hypertension to be a significant risk factor for the development of ischaemic heart disease, both independently and in association with other cardiovascular risk factors. Systolic hypertension has been shown to correlate positively with ischaemic heart disease across all ages. Systolic blood pressure as a risk factor for ischaemic heart disease in middle-aged and elderly populations should be interpreted in the context of diastolic blood pressure and pulse pressure.

The association between blood pressure and ischaemic heart disease has been shown to be continuous, with each increase in systolic blood pressure of 20 mmHg at least doubling the risk of death from ischaemic heart disease, alongside other vascular causes. Recent trials have found significant reduction in ischaemic heart disease risk with lower systolic blood pressure targets than the long-standing target of <140 mmHg, with some identifying a target systolic blood pressure of <130 mmHg as providing an optimal balance between ischaemic heart disease risk reduction and the risk of adverse events secondary to a patient's antihypertensive treatment.

5.3 Hypertension and stroke

Hypertension is the most prevalent risk factor for stroke, appearing in approximately 64% of patients with stroke. Blood pressure has been shown to have a continuous relationship with stroke (both ischaemic and haemorrhagic) across all ages. At midlife (ages 40–69), stroke risk more than doubles for each increase of 20 mmHg in systolic blood pressure or 10 mmHg in diastolic blood pressure in the range from 115/75 to 185/115 mmHg. Pulse pressure has not shown a correlation with stroke risk. As with ischaemic heart disease, recent trials have suggested a target systolic blood pressure of <130 mmHg after identifying a significant reduction in stroke risk with lower systolic blood pressure targets than the commonly used <140 mmHg.

In addition to a relationship with the incidence of both ischaemic and haemorrhagic stroke, hypertension has been shown to impact outcomes in both events. In haemorrhagic stroke, systolic hypertension has been associated with increased haematoma growth, mortality, and neurological deterioration. In patients with ischaemic stroke receiving intravenous thrombolysis, systolic hypertension has been associated with post-stroke intracerebral haemorrhage.

5.4 Hypertension and other cardiovascular risk factors—risk scoring

The Framingham Heart Study found a set of cardiovascular risk factors that tended to occur alongside one another, in a pattern that has since been termed 'metabolic clustering'. The Framingham study notes that, of those with hypertension, only 22% of men and 18% of women were hypertensive, independent of other cardiovascular risk factors. One additional cardiovascular risk factor was identified in almost 30% of hypertensive patients, and 50% of the hypertensive study participants were found to have two or more additional cardiovascular risk factors. The metabolic cardiovascular risk factors most commonly associated with hypertension are dyslipidaemias, elevated body mass index, and hyperglycaemia. The cardiovascular risk of these metabolic risk factors, with inclusion of smoking as an additional risk factor, is multiplicative.

Owing to this clustering of cardiovascular risk factors alongside hypertension, various models have been created to assess cardiovascular risk due to blood pressure in the context of these additional risk factors. Most systems aim to assess the 10-year risk of cardiovascular event. The European Society of Cardiology recommends use of the Systematic Coronary Risk Evaluation (SCORE) system, which interprets systolic blood pressure, along with age, gender, total cholesterol, smoking status, and location (Figures 5.1 and 5.2). An alternative is the QRISK3 cardiovascular risk assessment tool which takes into account a patient's diabetic status, along with numerous other risk factors not incorporated into the SCORE system, and is the recommended risk assessment tool in UK practice. Chapter 12 discusses in greater detail methods to lower this cardiovascular risk.

5.5 Diastolic hypertension

Through a variety of studies, including the Framingham Heart Study, systolic blood pressure has proven to be a better predictor of cardiovascular risk than diastolic blood pressure. However, diastolic blood pressure has also been shown to correlate with future cardiovascular risk in an age-dependent fashion. Increased peripheral resistance, caused by arterial vasoconstriction, is the cause of increased diastolic blood pressure. In early medical literature, hypertension was defined using diastolic blood pressure only.

In the Framingham Heart Study, in patients under the age of 50, diastolic hypertension has been shown to positively correlate with the metabolic syndrome and future cardiovascular risk. Conversely, above the age of 50, low diastolic blood pressure has been shown to increase the risk of further myocardial infarction and heart failure. Thus, diastolic pressure is negatively correlated with cardiovascular risk in middle-aged and elderly populations, whilst being positively correlated with cardiovascular risk for younger populations. This relationship is known as the J-curve and is a well-established phenomenon.

The relationship between diastolic hypertension and stroke is not well established across all ages. Both systolic hypertension and diastolic hypertension demonstrate a significant association with stroke risk in younger patients (aged 45 and less). However, above the age of 45, systolic hypertension serves as a better indicator of stroke risk, impacted by the age-associated decline in diastolic blood pressure secondary to arterial stiffening. Additionally, low diastolic blood pressure is not as established as a risk factor for stroke or renal disease as it is for

SCORE - European Low Risk Chart

10 year risk of fatal CVD in low risk regions of Europe by gender, age, systolic blood pressure, total cholesterol and smoking status

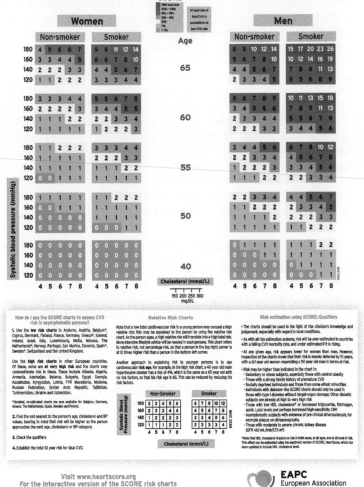

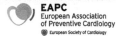

Figure 5.1 SCORE chart for low-risk countries.

Reproduced with permission from 'Estimation of ten-year risk of fatal cardiovascular disease in Europe: the SCORE project' *European Heart Journal*, Volume 24, Issue 11, 1 June 2003, Pages 987–1003, https://doi.org/10.1016/S0195-668X(03)00114-3. Available at: https://www.escardio.org/Education/Practice-Tools/CVD-prevention-toolbox/SCORE-Risk-Charts.

ischaemic heart disease. This is because the coronary arteries are perfused during diastole; thus, if the pressure is lower in the presence of significant stenoses, then the risk of ischaemia will be greater. This is not a factor for the cerebral or renal circulation where perfusion occurs mainly in systole.

Taken altogether, it is important to acknowledge the role of diastolic blood pressure in cardiovascular risk, despite the superiority of systolic hypertension as a predictor of future cardiovascular risk. In practical terms, this means taking a patient-centred approach when considering diastolic blood pressure, as the patient's age and comorbidities will have a great impact on what diastolic blood pressure targets should be.

5.6 Hypertension and left ventricular hypertrophy

Hypertension is an important cause of left ventricular hypertrophy (LVH). LVH has been shown in many studies to be a strong predictor of cardiovascular events. It is also widely regarded as a surrogate marker for other cardiovascular risk factors: age, smoking, obesity, and diabetes mellitus. The risk of cardiovascular events proportionally increases as left ventricular (LV) mass increases. As the left ventricle increases in size, the coronary reserve decreases and there is increased cardiac oxygen requirements. This can, in turn, give rise to ectopy, as well as impaired LV filling and contractility.

Encouragingly, numerous studies have identified a reduction in LV mass as a factor that can contribute to a decrease in future risk of cardiovascular events. The Losartan Intervention For Endpoint reduction in hypertension (LIFE) study consistently demonstrated that a greater reduction in LVH led to a greater reduction in cardiovascular risk. This gives physicians a clear treatment goal in these patients.

Patients with LVH are at an increased risk of sudden death from stroke, myocardial infarction, and ventricular arrhythmia. LVH is discussed in more detail in Chapter 6.

5.7 Hypertension and peripheral vascular disease

The presence of peripheral vascular disease (PVD) is a significant cardiovascular risk factor. Intermittent claudication, caused when blood flow is insufficient to meet the body's metabolic needs, is the most common symptomatic manifestation of PVD. The presence of claudication increases the risk of cardiovascular death 3- to 5-fold.

Roughly half of patients diagnosed with PVD will also have hypertension. Hypertension contributes to the pathogenesis of atherosclerosis through abnormalities in haemostasis and lipids, thus leading to an increased atherothrombotic state. The Framingham Heart Study documented a 2- to 4-fold increased risk of developing PVD with hypertension. Additionally, hypertension is clearly associated with aneurysmal disease, particularly abdominal aortic aneurysmal disease.

SCORE - European High Risk Chart

10 year risk of fatal CVD in high risk regions of Europe by gender, age, systolic blood pressure, total cholesterol and smoking status

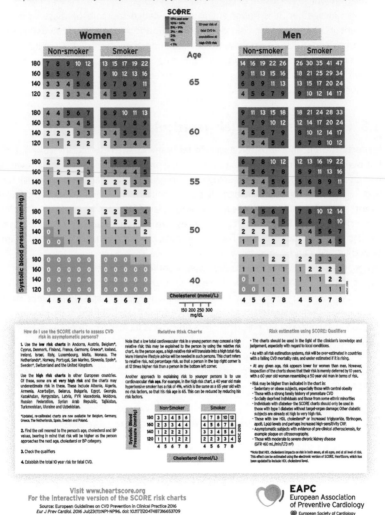

Figure 5.2 SCORE chart for high-risk countries.

Reproduced with permission from 'Estimation of ten-year risk of fatal cardiovascular disease in Europe: the SCORE project.' *European Heart Journal*, Volume 24, Issue 11, 1 June 2003, Pages 987–1003, https://doi.org/10.1016/S0195-668X(03)00114-3. Available at: https://www.escardio.org/Education/Practice-Tools/CVD-prevention-toolbox/SCORE-Risk-Charts.

CHAPTER 5

Atherosclerosis, particularly in the renal arteries, can self-perpetuate hypertension through activation of the renin–angiotensin–aldosterone system. Half of patients with PVD and hypertension will also have renal artery stenosis. This is an important consideration, as starting angiotensin-converting enzyme (ACE) inhibitor therapy for these patients can have a significant impact on renal function. More on the renin–angiotensin–aldosterone system and ACE inhibitors can be found in Chapter 17.

5.8 Conclusion

Hypertension is a significant risk factor for cardiovascular disease, and successful reduction of elevated blood pressure leads to reduced cardiovascular risk. Systolic hypertension is a better predictor of risk than diastolic hypertension, but diastolic blood pressure still plays a key role. This is particularly true for ischaemic heart disease and stroke. Owing to the tendency to occur in the context of other cardiovascular risk factors, hypertension must always be interpreted in the clinical context. Current best practice is to employ cardiovascular risk calculators such as the QRISK3 or SCORE systems. Following recent studies demonstrating a significant reduction in risk at lower systolic blood pressures, treatment goals are moving towards a target systolic blood pressure of <130 mmHg for optimal cardiovascular risk reduction.

KEY REFERENCES

Bangalore S, Toklu B, Gianos E, et al. (2017). Optimal systolic blood pressure target after SPRINT: insights from a network meta-analysis of randomized trials. *Am J Med* **130**:707–19.e8.

Böhm M, Ferreira JP, Mahfoud F, et al. (2020). Myocardial reperfusion reverses the J-curve association of cardiovascular risk and diastolic blood pressure in patients with left ventricular dysfunction and heart failure after myocardial infarction: insights from the EPHESUS trial. *Eur Heart J* **41**:1673–83.

Böhm M, Schumacher H, Teo KK, et al. (2018). Achieved diastolic blood pressure and pulse pressure at target systolic blood pressure (120–140mmHg) and cardiovascular outcomes in high-risk patients: results from ONTARGET and TRANSCEND trials. *Eur Heart J* **39**:3105–14.

Chen Z, Mo J, Xu J, et al. (2020). Effect of low diastolic blood pressure to cardiovascular risk in patients with ischemic stroke or transient ischemic attacks under different systolic blood pressure levels. *Front Neurol* **11**:356.

Forouzanfar MH, Liu P, Roth GA, et al. (2017). Global burden of hypertension and systolic blood pressure of at least 110 to 115 mmHg, 1990–2015. *JAMA* **317**:165–82.

Franklin SS, Gokhale SS, Chow VH, et al. (2015). Does low diastolic blood pressure contribute to the risk of recurrent hypertensive cardiovascular disease events?: the Framingham Heart Study. *Hypertension* **65**:299–305.

Hippisley-Cox J, Coupland C, Brindle P (2017). Development and validation of QRISK3 risk prediction algorithms to estimate future risk of cardiovascular disease: prospective cohort study. *BMJ* **357**:j2099. doi:10.1136/bmj.j2099.

Lip GYH, Coca A, Kahan T, *et al*. (2017). Hypertension and cardiac arrhythmias: a consensus document from the European Heart Rhythm Association (EHRA) and ESC Council on Hypertension, endorsed by the Heart Rhythm Society (HRS), Asia-Pacific Heart Rhythm Society (APHRS) and Sociedad Latinoamericana de Estimulación Cardíaca y Electrofisiología (SOLEACE). *Europace* **19**:891–911.

Murray CJL, Aravkin AY, Zheng P, *et al*. (2020). Global burden of 87 risk factors in 204 countries and territories, 1990–2019: a systematic analysis for the Global Burden of Disease Study 2019. *Lancet* **396**:1223–49.

National Institute for Health and Care Excellence (2019). CVD risk assessment and management. Available from: https://cks.nice.org.uk/topics/cvd-risk-assessment-man agement/references/

Vos T, Lim SS, Abbafati C, *et al*. (2020). Global burden of 369 diseases and injuries in 204 countries and territories, 1990–2019: a systematic analysis for the Global Burden of Disease Study 2019. *Lancet* **396**:1204–22.

CHAPTER 5

Left ventricular hypertrophy

Yuichiro Yano and Sunil K. Nadar

KEY POINTS

* Left ventricular hypertrophy (LVH) is a well-known complication of long-standing hypertension, with the duration and severity of high blood pressure contributing to its development.
* The renin–angiotensin–aldosterone system (RAAS) has been implicated as one of pathophysiological mechanisms in the development of LVH.
* The presence of LVH in hypertensive patients is a predictor for adverse health outcomes, including coronary heart disease, stroke, heart failure, and all-cause mortality.
* Regression of LVH with treatment of hypertension can lead to a corresponding reduction in cardiovascular risk.
* The pathological role of angiotensin II in the development of LVH suggests that agents targeting the RAAS may offer beneficial effects beyond blood pressure reduction, possibly by inhibiting intracardiac RAAS and, specifically, the tropic effects of angiotensin II on the myocardium.
* Antihypertensive agents acting on the RAAS appear to be best at regressing LVH and improving outcomes.

6.1 Introduction

Left ventricular hypertrophy (LVH) is an important manifestation of hypertensive-mediated organ damage (HMOD). A recent meta-analysis suggests that the prevalence of LVH varies from 36% to 41% of a pooled population of hypertensive patients. Its prevalence is similar in males and females. LVH is predominantly related to the duration of hypertension and the levels of elevated blood pressures. The pathophysiological mechanisms involved in LVH include general hypertrophy of the muscles in response to contracting against a high arterial pressure. In the initial stages, LVH is therefore a compensatory process that represents an adaptation to increased ventricular wall stress.

Higher systolic and diastolic pressures are both closely related to higher left ventricular (LV) mass and wall thickness, respectively, suggesting an influence of both volume and pressure overload on cardiac muscles. Overall, the presence of LVH substantially increases the risk of stroke, coronary heart disease, heart failure, and arrhythmias.

6.2 Diagnosis of left ventricular hypertrophy

Diagnosis of LVH is made by both electrocardiography (ECG) and echocardiographic examination. Table 6.1 lists the common criteria used for the diagnosis of LVH. As ECG is often the first test that is done in patients with hypertension, there is a need for good diagnostic criteria. However, none of these criteria are universally accepted, as evidenced by different clinical trials using different criteria for the diagnosis of LVH. None of the criteria that are currently used have a good sensitivity; however, they are fairly specific.

Table 6.1 ECG criteria for diagnosing LVH		Sensitivity (%)	Specificity (%)
	Criteria		
Cornell criteria	RaVL plus an S wave in V3 >2.8 mV in men or >2.0 mV in women	22	95
Cornell voltage–duration	Cornell voltage × QRS duration	95	50–60
Sokolow–Lyon criteria	S wave in V1 plus an R wave in V5 or V6 >3.5 mV or an R wave in V5 or V6 >2.6 mV	25	95
Gubner–Ungerleider criteria	R wave in I plus an S wave in III >2.5 mV	13	95
Romhilt–Estes scoring system	Excessive amplitude: 3 points (largest R or S wave in limb leads ≥20 mV, or S wave in V1 or V2 ≥30 mV, or R wave in V5 or V6 ≥30 mV) ST–T segment pattern of LV strain: 3 points (ST–T segment vector shifted in direction opposite to mean QRS vector) Left atrial involvement: 3 points (terminal negativity of P wave in V1 ≥1 mm with duration ≥0.04 s) Left axis deviation: 2 points (left axis ≥ −30° in frontal plane) Prolonged QRS duration: 1 point (≥0.09 s) Intrinsicoid deflection: 1 point (intrinsicoid deflection in V5 or V6 ≥0.05 s) Two thresholds in use: positive if ≥4 points or ≥5 points	50	95

Echocardiography continues to be the gold standard for the diagnosis of LVH, although other modalities of imaging, such as magnetic resonance imaging or computed tomography (CT) scanning, can be used for diagnosis.

LVH is diagnosed based on calculation of the LV mass. The LV end-diastolic dimension (LVEDD), interventricular septum thickness in diastole (IVSd) and posterior wall thickness in diastole (PWd) are measured when echocardiography is performed to estimate the LV mass. The LV mass (in grams) is calculated using the American Society of Echocardiography (ASE) formula: $0.8 \times \{1.04 \times [(IVSd + LVEDD + PWd)^3 - (LVEDD)^3]\} + 0.6$. The LV mass index is calculated as LV mass/body surface area (g/m^2), as recommended by the ASE/European Society of Cardiovascular Imaging (ESCVI). The LV mass index can also be calculated as LV mass indexed to height$^{2.7}$ ($g/m^{2.7}$). The LVH is defined as an increased LV mass index of ≥ 96 g/m^2 in females and ≥ 116 g/m^2 in males (and an LV mass index of ≥ 45 $g/m^{2.7}$ in females and ≥ 49 $g/m^{2.7}$ in males when the LV mass is indexed to height$^{2.7}$). In accordance with the ASE/ESCVI recommendation, the methodology for LV mass estimation and LVH is similar across racial/ethnic groups.

6.3 Pathophysiology and development of left ventricular hypertrophy

There are four distinct patterns of LV geometry in hypertension (Figure 6.1). Normal LV geometry is identified by a normal LV mass and a normal relation between the cavity size and the wall thickness such as relative wall thickness (RWT). Concentric remodelling is characterized by a normal LV mass, but an increased RWT (RWT >0.45). Eccentric LVH is characterized by a large LV size, but a normal RWT (RWT <0.45); it is related to the volume load and may be

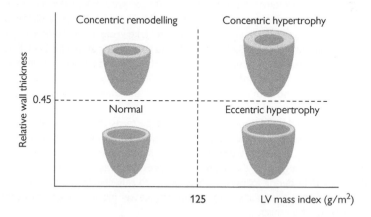

Figure 6.1 The four types of left ventricular geometry.

a physiological adaptation to dynamic exercise and is also common in obesity. Morphologically, eccentric LVH shows a relative increase in the number of myocytes. Concentric LVH occurs in conditions associated with pressure overload and is related to static exercise. LVH is a pathological condition with a relative increase in connective tissue and fibrosis often found in hypertension. In a pooled meta-analysis population, eccentric LVH was found to be the most common type of hypertrophy followed by concentric LVH.

Arterial pressure is the predominant haemodynamic factor and is usually the most powerful determinant of LV mass in hypertensive patients. However, the relatively low correlation coefficient between blood pressure and LV mass suggests that there are other mechanisms and factors that are equally, if not more, important. Other demographic determinants, such as age, race, sex, and body size, are all known to play a role in the development of LV mass.

Non-haemodynamic risk factors for the development of LVH include trophic factors mediated by the sympathetic nervous system, the renin–angiotensin–aldosterone system (RAAS), and insulin. Activation of the sympathetic nervous system has long been implicated in the development of LVH. Although in vitro studies appear to show a correlation between the two, in vivo studies have not been that definite. It also appears that LVH is related to the haemodynamic changes elicited by sympathetic nerve activation, rather than to a direct adrenergic effect on the myocardium.

Patients with LVH often have increased levels of insulin and insulin resistance. Insulin has trophic effects, and insulin resistance is more common among hypertensive patients than in normotensive subjects. Insulin resistance is associated with an attenuated therapeutic response to antihypertensive drugs. In contrast, the role of the RAAS in the development of LVH is much clearer. Circulating plasma levels of aldosterone and angiotensin II are related to the extent of LVH. It has been suggested that angiotensin II promotes myocyte cell growth and aldosterone may increase the collagen content and stimulate the development of myocardial fibrosis.

Leptin, a 16-kDa protein hormone that plays a key role in regulating energy intake and expenditure, has recently been found to be associated with LVH. Fasting plasma leptin levels are associated with LVH on echocardiography in human studies. In newly diagnosed hypertensive patients, higher fasting plasma leptin levels are associated with higher myocardial wall thickness, independently of 24-hour ambulatory blood pressure levels.

A study assessing 24-hour blood pressure patterns in 35 non-diabetic renal transplant recipients with versus those without LVH demonstrated that a lower nocturnal fall in blood pressure (non-dipper status) was associated with LVH. Another study suggested that higher pulse pressure was associated with an incidence of LVH during follow-up. Pulse pressure reflects the elasticity of blood vessels, and thus the mechanisms underlying vessel inelasticity and myocardial thickness may be similar.

The role of dietary salt in the pathogenesis of LVH was first described by Schmeider in 1988. Since then, others have also confirmed this to be true. It has

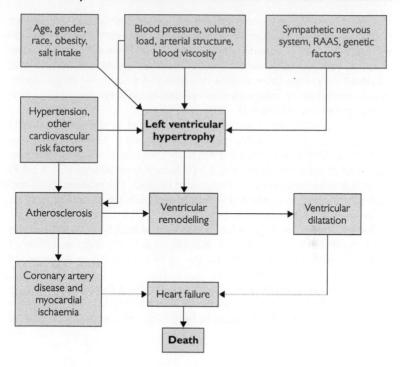

Figure 6.2 Complex correlations between hypertension, left ventricular hypertrophy, and cardiovascular morbidity and mortality.

been suggested that increased sodium intake increases the preload and thereby increases LVH. It has also been suggested to work via the RAAS and the sympathetic nervous system. The different aetiological factors are summarized in Figure 6.2.

LVH is also present in trained athletes, which is considered as a physiological adaptation (i.e. physiological LVH). This differentiation is required since physiological LVH is reversible and does not link to adverse prognosis, compared to pathological LVH. Although it is difficult to distinguish the two forms of LVH using ECG or echocardiography, physiological LVH may demonstrate normal diastolic filling patterns.

6.4 Prognostic aspects of hypertensive left ventricular hypertrophy

Casale and colleagues (1986) were among the first to demonstrate the relationship between adverse outcomes in hypertensive patients and LVH in a follow-up study of 140 men with uncomplicated hypertension over 5 years. Subsequent studies, including the Framingham Heart Study, have since demonstrated that LVH was associated with an increased risk of cardiovascular disease (CVD) events and all-cause mortality in community- and practice-based populations. For example, individuals with versus those without LVH have 2–4 times higher risk of cardio-vascular complications, independent of age, sex, blood pressure, smoking, cholesterol, and diabetes (Table 6.2).

LVH also predicts the development of stroke and atrial fibrillation. In the Framingham cohort, echocardiographic LVH was found to be predictive of incident stroke. After adjusting for other risk factors, the hazard ratio (HR) for stroke and transient ischaemic attack was 1.5 (95% confidence interval (CI) 1.2–1.8) for each quartile increment in height-adjusted LV mass. This relationship has also been demonstrated in a cohort of African Americans in the Atherosclerosis Risk in Communities (ARIC) study.

The development of atrial fibrillation in patients with LVH may be one pathway by which LVH can lead to strokes. For example, it has been shown that for every 1 standard deviation increase in LV mass, the risk of atrial fibrillation was increased by 1.2-fold.

LVH has also been associated with sudden cardiac death. Patients with LVH have an increased risk of ventricular arrhythmias after adjusting for other risk factors for ventricular ectopy. Predisposition to ventricular arrhythmias in LVH may be

Table 6.2 Studies demonstrating cardiovascular benefit with LVH regression

Authors, country, year	Subjects and methods	Findings
Muiesan, Italy, 1995	215 hypertensive patients (men and women) followed up for 10 years	More cardiovascular events in those without regression of LVH. In those with regression, the event rates were similar to the rates in those without baseline LVH
Verdecchia, Italy, 1998	430 hypertensive patients (men and women) followed up for 7–10 years	Event rate was 1.58 per 100 person years among those who achieved regression versus 6.27 among those who did not achieve LVH regression
Cipriano, France, 2001	474 hypertensive patients followed up for 5 years	Incidence of cardiovascular events was 4.8% in the group without LVH both before and during treatment, 9.6% in the group with LVH regression, and 15% in the group without regression of LVH
Koren, USA, 2002	172 patients followed up for 5 years	Event rate in those with LVH regression was 8.8%, and 19.8% in those without LVH regression

related to action potential prolongation, increased dispersion of refractoriness, and lowering of the ventricular fibrillation threshold.

Several mechanisms have been proposed to explain the increased cardiovascular risk associated with LVH. The most commonly proposed mechanism is that LVH serves as a surrogate marker for other risk factors. LVH is a measure of preclinical cardiac disease and is closely related to systemic atherosclerosis. It correlates with the carotid artery diameter and carotid intimal medial thickness. LVH is also associated with diastolic dysfunction as a result of myocardial fibrosis. This fibrosis may be mediated by angiotensin II.

The pattern of hypertrophy has clinical relevance. For example, concentric hypertrophy is more strongly associated with CVD events, compared to eccentric hypertrophy. The eccentric pattern of LV mass distribution reflects a normal extension to volume overload, whereas the concentric pattern reflects a response to pressure overload.

6.5 Treatment and regression of left ventricular hypertrophy

Lowering blood pressure leads to regression of LVH. Almost six decades ago, cardiac hypertrophy was shown to be reversed after nephrectomy in spontaneously hypertensive rats. At the same time, similar results were demonstrated in human hypertensive patients, with regression of LVH on ECG following blood pressure reduction. However, the clinical benefits with LVH regression have not been elucidated until recently. In general, few studies are powered sufficiently to detect the prognostic impact of serial changes of LVH either at ECG or echocardiography in hypertensive patients.

In the Framingham Heart Study, subjects with baseline LVH who showed an increase over time in ECG voltages were twice as likely to suffer a cardiovascular event over subsequent years, as compared to those with decreased voltages. A substudy of the Heart Outcomes Prevention Evaluation (HOPE) study (which compared the effects of ramipril, in addition to standard therapy, to placebo and vitamin E in about 9500 patients at high risk of cardiovascular events) demonstrated that the rate of stroke, heart attack, and cardiovascular death among those who did not develop LVH or experienced regression was 12.3%, whilst the rate was 15.8% among individuals who developed LVH or experienced no regression. The risk of developing congestive heart failure was 9.3% among participants who had regression or prevention of LVH, and 15.4% among those who had development or persistence of LVH.

Subsequently, there have been many studies showing that regression of LVH with treatment appears to decrease the chance of cardiovascular morbidity and mortality, and improves LV diastolic function (Table 6.2). A substudy from the Losartan Intervention For Endpoint reduction of hypertension (LIFE) study demonstrated that LVH regression, compared to no regression, was associated with lower admission rates for heart failure.

The effects on LVH regression by lowering blood pressure may differ by classes of antihypertensive agents as has been demonstrated by the LIFE study, as well as in a meta-analysis by Klingbeil and colleagues. This meta-analysis studied >80 trials with 146 active treatment arms (n = 3767 patients) and 17 placebo arms (n = 346 patients). After adjusting for various variables, there was a significant difference among the different medication classes. Use of angiotensin II receptor blockers (ARBs) decreased the LV mass index by 13%. There was a reduction in LV mass index by 11% with calcium antagonists, 10% with angiotensin-converting enzyme (ACE) inhibitors, 8% with diuretics, and 6% with beta blockers. In pairwise comparisons, ARBs, calcium antagonists, and ACE inhibitors were more effective at reducing LV mass index, compared to beta blockers.

Similar results have been obtained in the Prospective Randomized Enalapril Study Evaluating Regression of Ventricular Enlargement (PRESERVE) study and the Left Ventricular Hypertrophy Regression, Indapamide Versus Enalapril (LIVE) study. In the latter study, indapamide induced similar regression of LVH, as compared to enalapril. The meta-analysis by Klingbeil and colleagues suggested that direct vasodilators (such as hydralazine and minoxidil) may not cause LVH regression despite lowering blood pressure. This could be due to reflex stimulation of the RAAS, sympathetic nervous system, and other trophic hormone release, which may be directly involved in the development of LVH. Clonidine and prazosin may also be ineffective in LVH regression.

Recently, aldosterone blockade with spironolactone has also been shown to cause LVH regression. Similar findings were also noted with eplerenone, which caused similar reductions in LV mass, as compared to enalapril, but significantly higher reductions when the two drugs were combined.

Endothelin receptors are a new group of agents that are being studied in humans. Endothelin is known to be a vasoconstrictor and cause hypertension. It promotes growth of myocytes and collagen synthesis, which results in development of LVH. However, clinical trial data on its effect on reversing LVH are still awaited, but preliminary data are encouraging.

6.6 Optimal blood pressure levels for preventing development of left ventricular hypertrophy

Optimal blood pressure levels to prevent the development of LVH among hypertensive patients remain uncertain. In the Cardio-Sis study, an open-label randomized trial in Italy, non-diabetic patients with a systolic blood pressure of 150 mmHg or greater were randomly assigned to a target systolic blood pressure of <140 mmHg (usual control) or <130 mmHg (intensive control). The primary endpoint was the rate of ECG LVH 2 years after randomization. The incidence of LVH was lower in the intensive control group, compared to the usual control group (odds ratio 0.63; 95% CI 0.43–0.91; p = 0.013). In the Prevention of Hypertension in Patients with Pre-hypertension (PREVER–Prevention) trial, participants with pre-hypertension (systolic blood pressure 120–139 mmHg or diastolic blood pressure 80–89 mmHg) who were aged 30–70 years and did not reach optimal blood pressure after 3 months of lifestyle intervention were randomized to a chlorthalidone/amiloride combination pill or placebo. LV mass, assessed using Sokolow–Lyon voltage and voltage–duration product, decreased to a greater extent in participants allocated to the intervention group, compared to those in the placebo group. These results suggest that intensive versus usual blood pressure-lowering therapy may be of more benefit in preventing the development of LVH. The Systolic Blood Pressure Intervention Trial (SPRINT) suggested that, among individuals at high risk of CVD events but without diabetes mellitus (baseline mean systolic/diastolic blood pressure 140/78 mmHg), targeting systolic blood pressure of <120 mmHg, instead of <140 mmHg, resulted in a 36% lower rate of acute decompensated heart failure.

6.7 How does left ventricular hypertrophy regression translate into clinical outcomes?

The mechanisms underlying the association of changes in LV mass with clinical outcomes remain uncertain. As mentioned earlier, in hypertensive patients, LV mass and carotid intimal medial thickness correlate strongly. Therefore, with treatment, LVH regression could just be a surrogate marker for regression of atherosclerotic plaques.

Angiotensin II and angiotensin II type 1 receptor activation leads to proliferation of vascular smooth muscle cells and production of extracellular matrix protein, which result in the development of LVH and atherosclerosis. Furthermore, ARBs are the most potent at reducing LVH, supporting the effect of RAAS on the development of LVH.

Regression of LVH may occur through a reduction in myocyte volume and amount of interstitium. Studies showing regression of severe LVH after aortic valve replacement suggest an initial and rapid reduction in myocyte volume, followed by a continued reduction in interstitial fibrosis. This was demonstrated in a study of hypertensive patients using serial myocardial biopsies during treatment with lisinopril. There have also been studies demonstrating regression of LVH with salt restriction. Furthermore, a low-salt diet also appears to improve the LVH regression that is caused by antihypertensive agents.

6.8 Implications for hypertension management

Regression of LVH should be a target for treatment of hypertension. Except for minoxidil and hydralazine, most classes of hypertensive drugs have been shown to regress LVH. RAAS inhibitors and calcium channel blockers could reduce LV mass, independent of their blood pressure-lowering effect.

Regression of LVH in treated hypertensive patients should be considered as a favourable prognostic marker, which suggests a reduced risk of subsequent CVD.

In contrast, patients who have persistence or lack of regression of LVH over time should be considered at high cardiovascular risk, even in the presence of a normal achieved blood pressure. Intensive therapeutic management aimed at reducing blood pressure over a 24-hour period and strict control of concomitant modifiable risk factors are crucial to preventing LVH and CVD events.

KEY REFERENCES

Cuspidi C, Sala C, Negri F, et al. (2012). Prevalence of left-ventricular hypertrophy in hypertension: an updated review of echocardiographic studies. *J Hum Hypertens* **26**:343–9.

D'Ascenzi F, Fiorentini C, Anselmi F, Mondillo S (2021). Left ventricular hypertrophy in athletes: how to differentiate between hypertensive heart disease and athlete's heart. *Eur J Prev Cardiol* **28**(10):1125–33.

Klingbeil AU, Schneider M, Martus P, et al. (2003). A meta-analysis of the effects of treatment on left ventricular mass in essential hypertension. *Am J Med* **115**:41–6.

Lang RM, Badano LP, Mor-Avi V, et al. (2015). Recommendations for cardiac chamber quantification by echocardiography in adults: an update from the American Society of Echocardiography and the European Association of Cardiovascular Imaging. *J Am Soc Echocardiogr* **28**:1–39.e14.

Okin PM, Wachtell K, Gerdts E, et al. (2014). Relationship between left ventricular systolic function to persistence or development of electrocardiographic left ventricular hypertrophy in hypertensive patients: implications for the development of new heart failure. *J Hypertens* **32**:2472–8.

Papadopoulos A, Palaiopanos K, Protogerou AP, et al. (2020). Left ventricular hypertrophy and cerebral small vessel disease: a systematic review and meta-analysis. *Stroke* **22**:206–24.

Pewsner D, Jüni P, Egger M, et al. (2007). Accuracy of electrocardiography in diagnosis of left ventricular hypertrophy in arterial hypertension: systematic review. *BMJ* **335**:711.

Schmieder RE, Martus P, Klingbeil A (1996). Reversal of left ventricular hypertrophy in essential hypertension. A meta-analysis of randomized double-blind studies. *JAMA* **275**:1507–13.

Westaby JD, Miles C, Chis Ster I, et al. (2022). Characterisation of hypertensive heart disease: pathological insights from a sudden cardiac death cohort to inform clinical practice *J Hum Hypertens* **36**(3):246–53. doi:10.1038/s41371-021-00507-6

Yildiz M, Oktay AA, Stewart MH, et al. (2020). Left ventricular hypertrophy and hypertension. *Prog Cardiovasc Dis* **63**:10–21.

CHAPTER 6

CHAPTER 7

Atrial fibrillation and hypertension

Mohammed Najeeb Al-Rawahi

KEY POINTS

* Hypertension is considered to be an important risk factor for the development of atrial fibrillation.
* Left atrial changes in hypertension are thought to be responsible for the development of atrial fibrillation.
* Angiotensin-converting enzyme inhibitors and angiotensin receptor blockers appear to delay the development of atrial fibrillation in hypertensives.

7.1 Introduction

The prevalence of hypertension is growing, with 20–50% of the adult population worldwide being hypertensive. Hypertension and atrial fibrillation (AF) are related to an excess risk of cardiovascular disease and death. Because of its higher prevalence in the population, hypertension accounts for more cases of AF than other risk factors. In the Framingham study, hypertension was associated with an excess risk of AF by 50% in men and 40% in women, standing fourth after heart failure, ageing, and valvular heart disease. Similarly, in the Atherosclerosis Risk in Communities (ARIC) study, hypertension was the main contributor to the burden of AF, being responsible for 20% of new cases. Among patients with established AF, hypertension was present in 60–80% of individuals.

AF is becoming a growing burden to healthcare systems globally due to its morbidity and mortality. It is the most frequent cardiac arrhythmia in clinical practice, with 1–2% of the general population affected by the disease and 10% of individuals above the age of 75 diagnosed with AF. It is associated with a 5-fold increase in the risk of stroke, a 3-fold increase in the risk of congestive heart failure (CHF), and a 2-fold increase in mortality. The true prevalence of AF is likely higher than that indicated by current reports, as prolonged electrocardiographic monitoring will detect clinically silent AF in asymptomatic individuals.

Despite the well-established epidemiological association between hypertension and AF, the mechanisms explaining the higher tendency for hypertensive patients to develop AF are still incompletely known. The most robust animal and clinical contributory mechanisms will be discussed.

7.2 Hypertension and risk of atrial fibrillation

In the general population, hypertension increases the risk of AF in both sexes. In the Framingham Heart study, pulse pressure was superior to systolic blood pressure (SBP) and diastolic blood pressure (DBP) for prediction of AF, even after adjustment for left atrial (LA) dimension and left ventricular (LV) mass. Pulse pressure appeared as a significant independent risk factor for AF in patients with type 2 diabetes mellitus. Overall, these data suggest that arterial stiffness, reflected by pulse pressure, is an important and modifiable risk factor for AF development.

Thus, the majority of clinical studies showed a direct and linear relation between BP levels and the risk of AF. A post hoc analysis of the Ongoing Telmisartan Alone and in Combination With Ramipril Global Endpoint Trial (ONTARGET) and the Telmisartan Randomised Assessment Study in ACE Intolerant Subjects With Cardiovascular Disease (TRANSCEND) trial showed that the risk of AF significantly increased with systolic BP, pulse pressure, age, LV hypertrophy (LVH), body mass index, serum creatinine, and history of hypertension, and coronary and cerebrovascular disease. The impact of diastolic BP was not significant.

A blunted day–night fall in BP (non-dipping or reverse dipping pattern) is an independent predictor of major cardiovascular events and supraventricular and ventricular arrhythmias in hypertensive patients. In a study, hypertensive patients with a non-dipping pattern had a 2-fold higher risk of developing AF, when compared with those with a normal diurnal BP rhythm.

7.3 Pathophysiology

7.3.1 Morphological changes in the heart

In several animal models, hypertension has been shown to rapidly induce hypertrophy, fibrosis, and inflammation of the left atrium (LA). The main electrophysiological changes in the LA included enhanced heterogeneity of conduction with shortening of atrial wavelength and greater AF inducibility and duration. These electrophysiological abnormalities developed rapidly, being detectable just a few weeks after induction of hypertension by either banding of the ascending aorta or renal artery stenosis.

Human studies have also shown similar morphological changes in the heart of patients with hypertension. LA dilatation, along with LVH, are the most common and are associated with the duration of hypertension. Both LVH and LA dilatation are significant predictor of AF development, both in the general population and in hypertensive patients. Baseline LVH has been shown to double the risk of new-onset AF, with each 1 standard deviation increase in LV mass associated with a 20% (95% confidence interval (CI) 7–34%) increased risk of AF. Other changes in the atria of hypertensive patients include increased fibrosis and scarring within the atrial wall.

7.3.2 Role of the renin–angiotensin–aldosterone system

The renin–angiotensin–aldosterone system (RAAS) may be involved in the pathogenesis of AF through various mechanisms. These include proliferation of fibroblasts and extracellular matrix and hypertrophy of myocytes, with potentially unfavourable electrophysiological changes. Angiotensin II may also modulate some ion currents in myocytes, including the inward calcium (Ca^{2+}) current and the potassium current which promotes AF development. In isolated cardiac myocytes from rats and mice, angiotensin II activated cyclic adenosine monophosphate (cAMP)-dependent protein kinase A and Ca/calmodulin kinase II—a well-established proarrhythmogenic pathway in the setting of increased angiotensin II stimulation. Similarly, a 12-fold higher risk of AF has been reported in patients with primary hyperaldosteronism, when compared to patients with essential hypertension, which is in line with the known effect of aldosterone on cardiac inflammation, fibrosis, and hypertrophy. Several studies support the protective role of pharmacological RAAS inhibition against the risk of AF, which indirectly confirms the role of the RAAS in the causation of AF in hypertension.

7.4 Hypertension and atrial fibrillation in congestive heart failure

There is abundant evidence that hypertension is a major modifiable risk factor for CHF in terms of both heart failure with preserved ejection fraction (HFpEF) and heart failure with reduced ejection fraction (HFrEF). The prevalence of AF is 53% in HFrEF, and 65% in HFpEF. In patients with CHF, hypertension is a strong and independent predictor of AF, particularly when the ejection fraction (EF) is <50%. CHF remains the most common cause of death in patients with AF.

7.5 Treatment of atrial fibrillation in patients with hypertension

7.5.1 Intensive blood pressure control and risk of atrial fibrillation

The direct relation between high blood pressure (BP) and AF observed in epidemiological studies raises the possibility that non-pharmacological and pharmacological interventions, which delay progression from pre-hypertension to hypertension, may prevent the occurrence of new-onset AF. Similarly, intensive control of BP in hypertensive patients could decrease the risk of new-onset AF.

The recently published Systolic Blood Pressure Intervention Trial (SPRINT) enrolled participants with hypertension at increased risk of cardiovascular disease and randomized them to an intensive BP-lowering group (target SBP <120 mmHg), compared to standard BP lowering (target SBP <140 mmHg). A total of 8022 participants (4003 randomized to the intensive arm, and 4019 to the standard BP arm) who were free of AF at the time of enrolment were followed up for up to 5.2 years. Two hundred and six incident AF cases occurred—88 in the intensive BP-lowering arm, and 118 in the standard BP-lowering arm. Intensive BP lowering was associated with a 26% lower risk of developing new AF (hazard ratio (HR) 0.74, 95% CI 0.56–0.98; p = 0.037).

In the Studio Italiano Sugli Effetti Cardiovascolari Del Controllo Della Pressione Arteriosa Sistolica (Cardio-Sis) trial, 1111 patients with hypertension without diabetes mellitus, who were in sinus rhythm at entry, were enrolled and randomly assigned to a target SBP <140 mmHg (usual control) or <130 mmHg (tight control); new AF was a prespecified secondary outcome of the study. At the end of a median follow-up period of 2 years, new AF occurred in 3.8% of patients in the usual control group and in 1.8% of patients in the tight control group (HR 0.46, 95% CI 0.22–0.98; p = 0.044).

Therefore, intensive treatment of patients with hypertension to a target SBP of <120 mmHg has the potential to reduce AF development in follow-up.

7.5.2 Inhibition of the renin–angiotensin–aldosterone system and risk of atrial fibrillation

There are many animal, as well as human, studies that evaluated the effect of RAAS blockade (either by angiotensin-converting enzyme (ACE) inhibitors or angiotensin receptor blockers (ARBs)) in hypertensive subjects on the development of new-onset AF. As the RAAS has been implicated in the pathophysiology of the development of AF, it is only conceivable that its blockade would reduce the development of AF.

In the Studies of Left Ventricular Dysfunction (SOLVD) trial conducted in patients with LV systolic dysfunction (EF <35%), enalapril significantly reduced the risk of new-onset AF and this effect was independent of potential confounders. In other studies conducted in patients with severe CHF, candesartan (HR 0.80, 95% CI 0.65–0.99; p = 0.039) and valsartan (HR 0.63, 95% CI 0.49–0.81; p = 0.0003) were more effective than placebo in reducing new-onset AF. In the Trandolapril Cardiac Evaluation (TRACE) study—a comparison of trandolapril versus placebo in post-myocardial infarction patients with low EF—trandolapril significantly reduced the risk of new-onset AF by 55%.

Use of dual blockade of the RAAS with ACE inhibitors and ARBs in the ONTARGET/TRANSCEND trial in patients at high cardiovascular risk failed to decrease the incidence of new-onset AF in patients randomized to ramipril and telmisartan (6.8%), as compared to those randomized to telmisartan (6.9%) and ramipril (7.2%) alone.

In the Losartan Intervention for Endpoint reduction in hypertension (LIFE) study, the incidence of new-onset AF was 6.8 versus 10.1 per 1000 person-years of follow-up with losartan and atenolol, respectively (adjusted HR 0.67, 95% CI 0.55–0.83; p <0.001). In the Valsartan Antihypertensive Long-Term Use Evaluation (VALUE) study, valsartan reduced the incidence of new-onset AF in hypertensive patients, when compared to amlodipine-based therapy. In a small cohort of patients with persistent AF, irbesartan plus amiodarone were more effective than amiodarone alone in preventing AF recurrence after cardioversion.

In the Antihypertensive and Lipid-Lowering Treatment to Prevent Heart Attack Trial (ALLHAT), the incidence of new-onset AF did not differ significantly among the chlorthalidone (20.9 per 1000 patient-years), amlodipine (22.4 per 1000 patient-years), and lisinopril (20.6 per 1000 patient-years) groups, whereas it was higher in the doxazosin group. In a study from China, in which 149 hypertensive patients with paroxysmal AF were randomized to receiving either nifedipine or telmisartan, the rate of overall AF recurrence was similar in the two groups (59% with nifedipine and 55% with telmisartan), but the incidence of persistent AF was lower in the telmisartan group than in the nifedipine group (5.4% versus 16.0%; $p = 0.035$).

Overall, these studies suggest that inhibition of the RAAS with ACE inhibitors or ARBs might be considered for prevention of AF in hypertensive patients in sinus rhythm, although the evidence is not yet conclusive. The 2017 American College of Cardiology guidelines for management of hypertension suggested that ARBs can be useful for prevention of AF recurrence, with a class IIa recommendation.

7.6 Atrial fibrillation detection in high-risk subjects

Hypertensive patients who present in sinus rhythm with no prior history of AF and with clear evidence of cerebrovascular events—either an embolic ischaemic stroke or a transient ischaemic attack (TIA)—should be thoroughly investigated for AF, as many of them would have asymptomatic paroxysmal AF episodes. There are cardiac risk factors that make AF more plausible in such patients, including prior cryptogenic stroke, frequent palpitations, LV hypertrophy, LA dilatation, and being elderly.

Depending on the clinical characteristics of patients and the importance of making a diagnosis of silent AF, a progressive strategy may include frequent 12-lead electrocardiographic (ECG) screenings as a first step, followed by extended non-invasive ECG monitoring and eventually an implanted loop recorded.

7.7 Anticoagulation for atrial fibrillation

In patients with documented AF, hypertension increases the risk of thromboembolism and facilitates progression from paroxysmal to persistent or permanent AF. The prevalence of hypertension is similar in patients with asymptomatic and those with symptomatic AF.

The potential mechanisms linking hypertension with thromboembolism in patients with established AF are elusive. However, clinical studies suggest that hypertension could directly promote LA thrombosis, with hypertensive patients being shown to have a lower flow velocity and a higher risk of thrombosis in the LA appendage. Similarly, a subanalysis of the Stroke Prevention in Atrial Fibrillation III

(SPAF-III) study, demonstrated a significant inverse association between SBP and flow velocity in the LA appendage.

In a retrospective study from China, conducted in anticoagulated hypertensive patients with AF, those who achieved a target BP <130/80 mmHg showed a lower incidence of ischaemic stroke (0.9% versus 3.1% per year; $p = 0.01$), but a similar risk of major bleeding ($p = 0.61$) and intracranial bleeding ($p = 1.00$), when compared to patients with higher BP values.

Table 7.1 lists the different recommendations for anticoagulation in AF, and Figure 7.1 lists the algorithm for management. For an estimate of individual risk of stroke in AF patients, a history of hypertension contributes 1 point to the CHADS-65 (CHF, hypertension, age 65, diabetes mellitus, stroke (doubled)) score. The recent 2020 guidelines of the European Society of Cardiology (ESC) and the Canadian Cardiovascular Society (CCS) recommend anticoagulation for patients with hypertension and AF, regardless of age, preferably with a direct

Table 7.1 Assessment of risk of stroke in patients with atrial fibrillation through latest international guidelines

	2020 CCS AF guidelines	2020 ESC AF guidelines	2019 AHA/ACC/ HRS AF guidelines
Stroke risk score algorithm	CHADS2-65	CHA2DS2-VASc score	CHA2DS2-VASc score
Items (1 point each, except for stroke/TIA)	Age >65 Prior stroke or TIA Hypertension Heart failure Diabetes	Congestive heart failure Hypertension Age >75 Diabetes mellitus Stroke or TIA Vascular disease Age 65–74 Female	Congestive heart failure Hypertension Age >75 Diabetes mellitus Stroke or TIA Vascular disease Age 65–74 Female
OAC	Male ≥1 Female ≥1	Class Ia: Male ≥2 Female ≥3 Class IIa: Male = 1 Female = 2	Class I: Male ≥2 Female ≥3 Class IIb: Male = 1 Female = 2
Type of OAC	DOAC preferred over VKA	DOAC preferred over VKA	DOAC preferred over VKA

CCS, Canadian Cardiovascular Society; AF, atrial fibrillation; ESC, European Society of Cardiology; AHA, American Heart Association; ACC, American College of Cardiology; HRS, Heart Rhythm Society; TIA, transient ischaemic attack; OAC, oral anticoagulation; DOAC, direct oral anticoagulant; VKA, vitamin K antagonist.

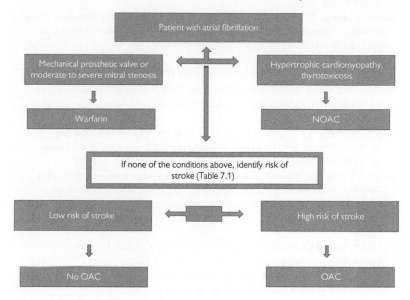

Figure 7.1 Anticoagulation in patients with atrial fibrillation.

oral anticoagulant (DOAC). The international guidelines recommend that pa-tients with AF with a 'CCS algorithm' (CHADS-65) score of 1 solely because of coexisting hypertension should be anticoagulated (ESC: class IIa, level of evidence B; CCS: strong recommendation, moderate quality).

7.8 Conclusion

Hypertension is the most important modifiable risk factor for AF. In patients with AF, management of hypertension is of paramount importance to pre-vent morbidity and mortality. Antihypertensive drugs that inhibit the RAAS might be preferred to reduce the risk of AF development, especially in pa-tients with LVF and CHF. DOACs are the preferred anticoagulation therapy in patients with hypertension and concomitant AF to prevent AF-related em-bolic stroke.

KEY REFERENCES

Andrade JG, Aguilar M, Atzema C, et al.; Members of the Secondary Panel (2020). The 2020 Canadian Cardiovascular Society/Canadian Heart Rhythm Society comprehensive guidelines for the management of atrial fibrillation. Can J Cardiol 36:1847–948.

Benjamin EJ, Levy D, Vaziri SM, D'Agostino RB, Belanger AJ, Wolf PA (1994). Independent risk factors for atrial fibrillation in a population-based cohort. The Framingham Heart study. JAMA 271:840–4.

Boriani G, Laroche C, Diemberger I, et al. (2015). Asymptomatic atrial fibrillation: clinical correlates, management, and outcomes in the EORP-AF Pilot General Registry. Am J Med 128:509–18.e2.

Fauchier L, Villejoubert O, Clementy N, et al. (2016). Causes of death and influencing factors in patients with atrial fibrillation. Am J Med 129:1278–87.

Freedman B, Camm J, Calkins H, et al.; AF-Screen Collaborators (2017). Screening for atrial fibrillation: a report of the AF-SCREEN International Collaboration. Circulation 135:1851–67.

Hindricks G, Potpara T, Dagres N, et al. (2021). 2020 ESC Guidelines for the diagnosis and management of atrial fibrillation developed in collaboration with the European Association of Cardio-Thoracic Surgery (EACTS). Eur Heart J 42, 373–498.

January CT, Wann LS, Alpert JS, et al.; ACC/AHA Task Force Members (2014). 2014 AHA/ACC/HRS guideline for the management of patients with atrial fibrillation: executive summary: a report of the American College of Cardiology/American Heart Association Task Force on practice guidelines and the Heart Rhythm Society. Circulation 130:2071–104.

Kirchhof P, Benussi S, Kotecha D, et al. (2016). 2016 ESC guidelines for the management of atrial fibrillation developed in collaboration with EACTS. Eur Heart J 37:2893–962.

Lau YF, Yiu KH, Siu CW, Tse HF (2012). Hypertension and atrial fibrillation: epidemiology, pathophysiology and therapeutic implications. J Hum Hypertens 26:563–9.

Seccia TM, Caroccia B, Adler GK, Maiolino G, Cesari M, Rossi GP (2017). Arterial hypertension, atrial fibrillation, and hyperaldosteron-ism: the triple trouble. Hypertension 69:545–50.

Soliman EZ, Rahman AKMF, Zhang Z-M, et al. (2020). Effect of intensive blood pressure lowering on the risk of atrial fibrillation. Hypertension 75:1491–6.

CHAPTER 8

The brain in hypertension

Arunodaya R. Gujjar

KEY POINTS

* Hypertension is a major risk factor for stroke and dementia.
* Large artery atherosclerosis and cerebral small vessel disease (CSVD) are considered to be a more direct consequence of chronic hypertension.
* Magnetic resonance imaging findings of white matter hyperintensities, lacunar infarcts, cerebral micro-bleeds, and brain atrophy are considered hallmark findings of CSVD.
* Early and prompt treatment of hypertension has been shown to prevent stroke and delay the onset of cognitive impairment in the elderly.

8.1 Introduction

The prevalence of hypertension increases with advancing age, which also corresponds to an increasing prevalence of several vascular and neurocognitive disorders. Stroke is the second most common cause of mortality in most developed countries and the most common cause of long-term disability. Dementia and cognitive disorders are common with increasing age and have a prevalence of around 5% at 60 years, which increases to >50% at 90 years. Hypertension is a significant, independent risk factor of both these conditions.

This chapter summarizes the relationship between hypertension and common neurovascular and neurocognitive disorders, reviewing the relevant pathophysiology, the evidence implicating hypertension in these conditions, and their clinical and management implications.

8.2 Hypertension and the brain: clinical syndromes

Hypertension is often asymptomatic in most individuals through most of its course. However, neurological involvement exemplifying 'end-organ damage' is well recognized in its varied manifestations (Box 8.1). Whilst acute changes in hypertension may directly influence neurological functioning, chronic hypertension causes neurological dysfunction mainly by contributing to age-associated vascular changes, as well as neurodegenerative processes.

> **Box 8.1** Clinical neurological syndromes associated with, and influenced by, hypertension
>
> 1. Syndromes directly associated with an acute increase in blood pressure:
>   a. Malignant hypertension
>   b. Eclampsia
>   c. 'Posterior reversible encephalopathy syndrome'
>   d. Hypertensive intracerebral haemorrhage
> 2. Neurological syndromes associated with/influenced by chronic, uncontrolled hypertension:
>   a. Large artery ischaemic stroke
>   b. Cerebral small vessel disease:*
>   i. Lacunar stroke
>   ii. Intracerebral haemorrhage
>   iii. Vascular dementia
>   iv. Vascular parkinsonism
>   c. Neurodegenerative disorders associated with vascular disease:*
>   i. Mild cognitive impairment
>   ii. Mood disorders
>   iii. Movement disorders/gait disorders
>   iv. Alzheimer's disease
>
> * (b) and (c) have overlapping syndromes.

Acute exacerbation of hypertension may manifest predominantly with neurological symptoms in the syndrome of hypertensive encephalopathy—with symptoms ranging from headache, blurred vision, seizures, and altered mental status to coma. Imaging correlates of this condition may include brain oedema, white matter hyperintensities (WMHs), or rarely ICH. A wide range of differential diagnosis may need to be considered in such patients, including neuroinfection, stroke, epilepsy, central nervous system (CNS) vasculitis, cerebral venous thrombosis, eclampsia, autoimmune encephalopathy, etc. (Hypertensive emergencies and related conditions are discussed in greater detail in Chapter 20.) *Chronic hypertension* is associated with two major neurological conditions as an independent risk factor—stroke and dementia, which are discussed here.

With advancing technology and, in particular, magnetic resonance imaging (MRI), Doppler ultrasound scanning, functional MRI, and positron emission tomography (PET) scanning, there has been an increasing awareness of the influence of hypertension on the brain, leading to the recognition of several preclinical changes. Despite such advances, major gaps do exist in the understanding of the pathophysiology and role of hypertension in these conditions.

CHAPTER 8

8.3 Stroke and hypertension

Unlike coronary artery disease, stroke is a heterogeneous condition. The two major types are ischaemic stroke and intracranial haemorrhage. Ischaemic stroke further includes subtypes recognized mainly by the underlying mechanism (as in the Trial of ORG 10172 in Acute Stroke Treatment (TOAST) and other classifications) as: large artery stroke, cerebral small vessel disease (CSVD), cardioembolism, and mixed/other mechanisms. Intracranial haemorrhage includes intracerebral (ICH) and subarachnoid haemorrhage.

Despite such heterogeneity, hypertension is a recognized risk factor and a major pathogenetic contributor to all subtypes of stroke, although to a somewhat variable extent. The pathogenetic mechanisms of these various types of stroke and their relation to hypertension (discussed in the sections below) also show a significant overlap. There is indeed great variability in the clinical manifestations of the various cerebrovascular pathologies, probably best exemplified by CSVD— which may cause ischaemic stroke and ICH, as well as cognitive impairment in different patients. Further different types of cerebrovascular diseases may coexist in the same patient, further complicating management issues.

8.3.1 Hypertension and large artery stroke

Large artery strokes are typified by those due to severe stenosis or occlusion of major cerebral arteries, for example, carotid, vertebral, basilar, or cerebellar arteries, components of the circle of Willis. These strokes typically occur due to atherosclerotic focal narrowing of the artery, sometimes complicated by focal thrombosis, artery-to-artery embolism, or less commonly arterial dissection. Such strokes usually injure large parts of the brain and hence are associated with greater morbidity and mortality.

Hypertension is a significant and independent risk factor for atherosclerosis, leading to stroke. Several other mechanisms have also been proposed to mediate cerebrovascular dysfunction due to the effect of chronic hypertension. Stiffening of large- and medium-sized arteries is a known consequence of chronic hypertension. This results in wider pulse pressure, enhanced reflected pressure waves from downstream impedence vessels, and greater shear force on the endothelium. Enhanced pulsatility has also been proposed to induce changes in brain microcirculation (another example of overlapping pathogenesis) such as remodelling of microcirculation, enhanced arteriolosclerosis, and changes in blood–brain barrier integrity and possible dysfunction. This has been proposed to contribute to CSVD (see Section 8.3.3), as well as having a possible direct neurodegenerative influence. Chronic hypertension is also known to shift the cerebral autoregulation curve to the right. The shape of the curve may also be altered. Studies, however, have shown that despite such shift, among subjects with essential hypertension, the actual cerebral blood flow does not change. The fact that control of hypertension has been repeatedly documented in prospective trials to lead to significant reduction in stroke recurrence does substantiate the role of hypertension in large artery stroke.

8.3.2 Hypertension and cardioembolism

Cardioembolic strokes essentially occur due to occlusion of a cerebral artery by a clot dislodged from the heart. Such strokes often occlude a major artery and hence are associated with the highest morbidity and mortality among ischaemic strokes. Hypertension appears to be related to cardioembolism indirectly through its relation to atrial fibrillation (AF), the most common cause of cardioembolism. Hypertension is an important risk factor for AF—those with hypertension are noted to have a 1.7-fold higher risk of AF, and consequently of stroke. Prompt and adequate management of hypertension is important in the management of patients with AF for prevention and rhythm control, as well as for control of heart failure.

8.3.3 Hypertension and cerebral small vessel disease

CSVD is recognized to be a dynamic whole-brain disorder, with an increasing prevalence as age advances. Two major types of CSVD are recognized: hypertensive arteriolosclerosis (or hypertensive CSVD) and cerebral amyloid angiopathy (CAA). Hypertensive CSVD is responsible for about a quarter of all ischaemic strokes and for 80% of all ICH. Hypertension is the most important risk factor for this variety, whereas diabetes mellitus, smoking, and hyperlipidaemia may contribute to a lesser extent. Hypertensive CSVD mainly causes angiopathy and parenchymal changes concentrated in the basal ganglia and deep cerebral white matter, as well as the pons. In contrast, CAA is characterized by deposition of amyloid beta peptide in the walls of arterioles and capillaries, mainly in the cerebral cortex and leptomeninges, leading to vascular injury and consequences rather similar to those of hypertensive CSVD. CAA is considered a manifestation of ageing and a degenerative condition, with hypertension and diabetes mellitus being less significant risk factors than for hypertensive CSVD. CAA almost always accompanies Alzheimer's disease and may mediate some of its pathology. Both hypertensive CSVD and CAA have similar pathological, imaging, and clinical manifestations, but differ in their predominant distribution in the brain—although with some overlap recognized.

8.3.3.1 Pathogenesis of cerebral small vessel disease

Damage to small arteries and arterioles causing cerebral infarcts was first documented in detail and elaborated by Miller Fisher in 1982. The microcirculation in the CNS is distinct from peripheral circulation in that it has a 'blood–brain barrier' which tightly controls the transfer of various metabolites into or out of the brain interstitial space—so as to preserve a stable internal milieu for neurons to function in. The 'neurovascular unit', as described in Figure 8.1, is recognized to be the structural basis of the blood–brain barrier. Changes in the neurovascular unit are believed to be central to the pathogenesis of both CSVD, as well as components

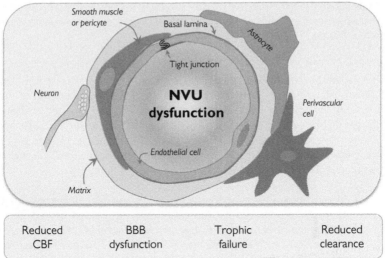

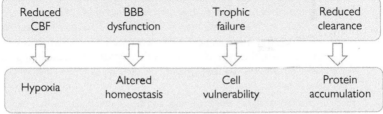

Figure 8.1 Illustration depicting the components of the neurovascular unit, which constitutes the 'blood–brain barrier', and the mechanisms of neuronal injury. Endothelial cells with tight junctions line the microvessels and are surrounded by a basement membrane, outside which are smooth muscle cells, pericytes, and the foot processes of astrocytes. The distal processes of these astrocytes are located near synapses or neurons. This entire unit functions dynamically to regulate the movement of nutrients, fluids, electrolytes, respiratory gases, neurotransmitter metabolites, etc. Neurovascular unit injury or dysfunction is implicated in cerebral small vessel disorders.

NVU, neurovascular unit; CBF, cerebral blood flow; BBB, blood–brain barrier.

Reproduced with permission from Iadecola C. The Neurovascular Unit Coming of Age: A Journey through Neurovascular Coupling in Health and Disease. Neuron. 2017;96(1):17–42. https://doi.org/10.1016/j.neuron.2017.07.030.

of neurodegeneration. The complex interaction of age with hypertension, as well as a myriad of other risk factors, has been proposed to cause a variety of pathological changes, including remodelling of arterioles, myogenic reactivity, hypertrophy, endothelial dysfunction, etc., which, in turn, may lead to ischaemia, exposure to toxic chemicals normally excluded from the brain interstitium, demyelination, decreased potential for remyelination, ischaemic injury, and loss of neural tissue. These microvascular changes may also be associated with deposition of amyloid beta in the vascular walls (typical of CAA and Alzheimer's disease).

As mentioned earlier, hypertension may also injure the cerebral microcirculation through large artery stiffening and transmission of higher pressure waves in to the cerebral tissue.

8.3.3.2 How to recognize cerebral small vessel disease?

The cerebral microcirculation cannot be examined easily by imaging. On MRI, CSVD is inferred by the presence of several changes considered typical of this condition, and which have evolved to be the most commonly reported incidental changes on MRI performed in the elderly. Five per cent of asymptomatic adults at 50 years have such changes, whilst this increases to about 90% at 90 years of age. The following is a brief description of typical MRI changes due to CSVD, with a brief description of their clinical implications:

- WMHs: these are lesions of variable size (thought to occur due to damage to myelin secondary to microvascular ischaemia or blood–brain dysfunction) in the cerebral white matter (sometimes also in the brainstem or cerebellum) which are hyperintense in T2 or fluid-attenuated inversion recovery (FLAIR) MRI sequences. Often asymptomatic, but when present in large numbers, they are associated with a higher-than-doubled risk of ischaemic stroke and a 3-fold greater risk of ICH, as well as a significant risk of dementia.

- Lacunar infarcts: these are small infarcts (1.5–2 cm in size) with a round, oval, or fluted shape, likely consequent to parenchymal ischaemia in the territory supplied by a small penetrating artery (although other mechanisms have also been proposed). Lacunar infarcts account for up to 25% of all ischaemic strokes. They are associated with a significant higher risk of future stroke and ICH, as well as cognitive decline.

- Cerebral micro-bleeds (CMBs): these are small microscopic foci of haemosiderin deposited around possibly leaky arterioles affected by fibrinoid necrosis or aneurysmal changes in the wall. These are typically well seen as focal hypointensities on susceptibility-weighted images (SWIs) on MRI, usually with a bloom effect (i.e. they appear larger than they actually are). CMBs are considered clinically asymptomatic, although they are the lesions preceding ICH. When numerous (>10), they may also confer a higher risk of ICH in the context of intravenous thrombolysis with recombinant tissue plasminogen activator (rtPA) administered for incidental acute ischaemic stroke.

- ICH: these are overt parenchymal haematomas due to disintegration of a small penetrating artery as a consequence of either CSVD or CAA; 80% of all cases of ICH are attributable to hypertensive CSVD, and the remainder to CAA. Typically, hypertensive ICH is located in the basal ganglia, thalamus, or brainstem.

• Brain atrophy: this is recognized to be a consequence of small vessel disease of any denomination and marks the neurodegenerative influence of chronic hypertension.

The above MRI manifestations of CSVD, when recognized among adults and older individuals, are consistently and strongly associated with a high incidence of ischaemic and haemorrhagic strokes, dementia, and depression, as well as all-cause mortality.

8.4 Hypertension and neurocognitive/ neurodegenerative disorders

Advancing age is associated with a range of neurocognitive and neurodegenerative changes through various mechanisms. Hypertension is now known to influence most mechanisms to variable extent. Among these conditions, minimal (or mild) cognitive impairment (MCI) and dementia are the most important because of their high prevalence and major influence on quality of life. MCI refers to a condition where mild changes in memory, language functions, attention, judgement, and complex decision-making are noticeable but do not significantly impair daily functioning. Such symptoms though are considered a prelude to dementia and may also occur due to many treatable conditions such as depression, nutritional deficiencies, endocrine dysfunction, and dehydration.

Numerous studies— both cross-sectional and longitudinal–have demonstrated that hypertension is associated with an increased risk of MCI, vascular dementia, and Alzheimer's disease. The importance of this observation is that hypertension is possibly one treatable risk factor, of which effective control may result in prevention of a significant proportion of the two major causes of dementia in the population. Similarly to the Framingham study alluded to earlier, several studies have demonstrated a relation between mid-life hypertension and cognitive decline, incident MCI, and dementia. These studies emphasize that the effect of hypertension in mid life is most pronounced in late-life cognitive decline. Among adults with MCI, uncontrolled hypertension is associated with a greater risk of progression to dementia. Components of blood pressure, such as increased systolic or diastolic blood pressure, pulse pressure, blood pressure variability, and postural hypotension, are all associated with an increased risk of cognitive decline. Some studies have demonstrated a U-shaped relationship between cognition and blood pressure, with greater dysfunction observed among subjects with a blood pressure >160 mmHg or a systolic blood pressure <130 mmHg. However, this is mostly limited to elderly subjects only. The course of the blood pressure profile over an individual's lifetime may also influence the risk of cognitive decline. In the Honolulu-Asia Aging Study (HAAS), cognitive decline was worse among those elderly subjects who had experienced a recent decline in blood pressure over the previous few years. A confounding issue concerning this study is that such late decline in blood pressure may be a consequence of dementia, rather than its cause.

The greatest impact among patients with long-standing hypertension appears to be on executive function, motor speed, and attention—domains which are more typical of 'subcortical' dementia such as vascular dementia. However, the difficulties in diagnosing the cause of dementia and the frequent overlap between the two major types often have limited such studies.

The mechanisms by which uncontrolled chronic hypertension influences cognitive and functional decline have been extensively explored. These are similar to those described in the pathogenesis of large artery, as well as small vessel, disorders discussed earlier. The major impact of such changes on the brain appears to be through parenchymal changes typical of CSVD—WMHs, lacunar infarcts, ICH, micro-bleeds, dilated perivascular spaces, and brain atrophy. Despite the strong association between mid- and late-life hypertension and cognitive decline, it is not entirely clear whether this effect is mediated predominantly through its effect on the cerebral vasculature or whether it also independently influences the neuropathology of Alzheimer's disease. Some of the evidence supporting a possible direct influence of chronic hypertension on Alzheimer's disease are the observation that chronic hypertension is associated with a higher late-life brain load of amyloid beta, higher tau protein deposition, and greater atrophy of the hippocampus on MRI.

8.5 Therapeutic implications

Acknowledging the strong relationship between hypertension and the risk of all cerebrovascular disorders, prompt and effective control of hypertension is recommended by all guidelines at all stages of life, aimed at primary and secondary prevention. The beneficial effect of prevention of cerebrovascular events appears to be attributable to the overall reduction in blood pressure, rather than specific agents utilized for this purpose.

Given the very limited methods available currently to treat or prevent the most common types of dementias, and the known relationship between chronic hypertension and the risk of dementia, control of hypertension appears to be a favourable and appealing target. Several studies have documented the beneficial effect of controlling hypertension on cognitive decline. In the Epidemiology of Vascular Ageing (EVA) study, treatment of hypertension for even 4 years translated to reduced cognitive decline, compared to untreated hypertension. Further longer duration of treatment has been shown to be associated with a greater reduction in the risk of dementia, with the greatest reduction being noted in individuals treated for >12 years' duration. Overall, treatment of hypertension results in a greater risk reduction for vascular dementia, in contrast to Alzheimer's disease.

The role of other vascular risk factors is also important in the risk of cognitive decline. Hypertension in the context of diabetes mellitus, hyperlipidaemia, and a higher waist-to-hip ratio has been shown to be associated with worse cognitive decline than hypertension alone. Control of such risk factors would also be important in ensuring the efficacy of antihypertensive treatment in the prevention of dementia.

Whether one class or a specific antihypertensive agent is more effective than others in the prevention of cognitive decline is as yet controversial. Although most agents have been shown to be effective in preventing cognitive decline, blockers of the renin–angiotensin–aldosterone system have been shown to be more effective than others in head-to-head comparisons.

8.6 Conclusion

Hypertension is an established risk factor for many neurological conditions such as stroke and dementia. Many changes in the brain are present in patients with hypertension, even before they become clinically relevant. In the above context, early recognition and prompt and adequate treatment of hypertension are important in the prevention of stroke and dementia. Despite recent advances, many gaps remain in our understanding of the pathogenetic concepts in the role of hypertension as a risk factor for dementia.

KEY REFERENCES

Anonow WS (2017). Hypertension and cognitive impairment. *Ann Transl Med* 5:259.

Bryan Williams B, Mancia G, Spiering W, *et al.*; ESC Scientific Document Group (2018). 2018 ESC/ESH Guidelines for the management of arterial hypertension. *Eur Heart J* 39:3021–104.

Gujjar AR, El-Tigani M, Lal D, Kakaria AK, Al-Asmi AR (2018). Different strokes: a management dilemma. *Sultan Qaboos Univ Med J* 18:e202–7.

Gujjar AR, Nandhagopal R, Jacob PC, *et al.* (2015). Ischemic stroke outcomes in Oman: experience of a university-hospital based stroke registry. *J Neurol Sci* 357:e380.

Iadecola C, Gottesman RF (2019). Neurovascular and cognitive dysfunction in hypertension: epidemiology, pathobiology, and treatment. *Circ Res* 124:1025–44.

Iadecola C, Yaffe K, Biller J, *et al.* (2016). Impact of hypertension on cognitive function: a scientific statement from the American Heart Association. *Hypertension* 68:e67–94.

Lennon MJ, Makkar SR, Crawford JK, Sachdev PS (2019). Midlife hypertension and Alzheimer's disease: a systematic review and meta-analysis. *J Alzheimer Dis* 2019;71:307–16.

McGrath ER, Beiser AS, DeCarli C, *et al.* (2017). Blood pressure from mid- to late life and risk of incident dementia. *Neurology* 89:2447–54.

Petrea RE, O'Donnell A, Beiser AS, *et al.* (2020). Mid to late life hypertension trends and cerebral small vessel disease in the Framingham Heart Study. *Hypertension* 76:707–14.

Rensma SP, van Sloten TT, Launer LJ, Stehouwer CDA (2018). Cerebral small vessel disease and risk of incident stroke, dementia and depression, and all-cause mortality: a systematic review and meta-analysis. *Neurosci Biobehav Rev* **90**:164–73.

Turana Y, Tengkawan J, Chia YC, *et al.* (2019). Hypertension and dementia: a comprehensive review from the HOPE Asia Network. *J Clin Hypertens* **21**:1091–8.

Walker KA, Power MC, Gottesman RF (2017). Defining the relationship between hypertension, cognitive decline, and dementia: a review. *Curr Hypertens Rep* **19**:1–16.

CHAPTER 8

CHAPTER 9

The kidneys in hypertension

Sarah Ahmad and Jordana B. Cohen

KEY POINTS

- Chronically and acutely elevated blood pressures can cause damage to the kidneys due to impaired or overwhelmed kidney autoregulation.
- Progression of chronic kidney disease from inadequate blood pressure control occurs due to several mechanisms, including micro- and macrovascular injury from barotrauma and neurohormonal dysregulation.
- Stringent and consistent blood pressure control is the most effective way to reduce the risk of progression of chronic kidney disease due to hypertension.

9.1 Introduction

There is a bidirectional relationship between hypertension and chronic kidney disease. Much like several other organs, the kidney is susceptible to microvascular and macrovascular damage as a result of both acutely elevated blood pressures and inadequate control of chronic hypertension. Kidney autoregulatory mechanisms help to mitigate microvascular injury from elevations in blood pressure in healthy individuals, but can become impaired or overwhelmed, leaving the kidney unprotected. Whilst the causal relationship of hypertension with incident chronic kidney disease is controversial, ample evidence supports the relationship of inadequate blood pressure control with progression of chronic kidney disease. Here we examine the physiological and epidemiological evidence related to kidney target organ injury in hypertension, as well as clinical approaches to try to minimize adverse renal effects from elevated blood pressure.

9.2 Overlying mechanisms of the effect of hypertension on the kidney as a target organ

Chronic hypertension may elicit organ damage by means of neurohormonal dysregulation causing unregulated vasoconstriction. Elevated blood pressures over many years can damage several organs as a result of the direct effects of blood pressure on the vasculature of those organs. The causal association of chronic elevation in blood pressure with the incidence of chronic kidney disease is controversial. Nonetheless, high-quality evidence supports the fact that chronically elevated blood pressure hastens the rate of progression of chronic kidney disease. Additionally, sudden and severe elevations in blood pressure can cause kidney microangiopathy and organ failure.

9.2.1 Hypothesized pathophysiological effect of chronic hypertension on the kidneys

In the setting of chronically elevated blood pressure, upregulation of the renin–angiotensin system and sympathetic tone as well as dysfunctional pressure and natriuresis promote intrarenal vasoconstriction that likely ultimately leads to focal global and segmental glomerulosclerosis. Due to intrarenal renin activation, the remaining glomeruli also undergo hyperfiltration, causing proteinuria, propagating focal segmental glomerular sclerosis and ultimately leading to renal fibrosis (Table 9.1).

Renal autoregulatory mechanisms (i.e. myogenic response and tubuloglomerular feedback) are primarily responsible for preventing damage to the renal vascular bed by protecting against shear stress and vascular barotrauma. In patients with hypertension, these mechanisms are thought to be impaired or overwhelmed, leading to chronic vascular damage. In normal states, the rapid myogenic response and more delayed tubuloglomerular feedback manipulate the afferent arteriole to maintain the preglomerular blood

Table 9.1 Clinical and pathological abnormalities observed due to kidney target organ damage in hypertension

Target of hypertensive damage	Abnormal finding potentially seen on clinical monitoring	Pathological abnormalities potentially seen on kidney biopsy
Kidney parenchymal disease	• Elevated serum creatinine or cystatin C • Microalbuminuria	• Focal global glomerulosclerosis • Focal segmental glomerulosclerosis • Interstitial fibrosis • Tubular atrophy • Glomerular necrosis
Vascular disease	• Elevated serum creatinine or cystatin C • Microalbuminuria • Haematuria • Renal artery stenosis on Doppler ultrasound, computed tomography angiography, or magnetic resonance angiography • Arteriosclerosis on computed tomography arteriography	• Atherosclerotic renal artery disease • Microangiopathy • Hyalinosis • Thrombotic microangiopathy • Endarteritis • Arteriolitis

flow and glomerular filtration rate within a range of perfusion pressure that prevents barotrauma. The myogenic response occurs when the vascular smooth muscle cells are stretched, leading to a cascade of intracellular signalling and intracytosolic calcium that result in vasoconstriction. The macula densa tubuloglomerular feedback response occurs when there is a rise in renal perfusion pressure causing decreased proximal tubular reabsorption of sodium, which results in a higher sodium load being delivered to the macula densa cells and leads to vasoconstriction of the adjacent afferent arteriole. These mechanisms decrease the preglomerular hydrostatic pressure. In the absence of adequate renal autoregulation (i.e. in hypertensive states and chronic kidney disease), the kidney is thought to be susceptible to barotrauma from the effects of elevated blood pressures on the normally protected microvasculature.

The pathological renal lesions observed in patients with chronic kidney disease thought to be related to hypertension are characterized by vasculopathy, glomerulopathy, and interstitial inflammation and fibrosis. Intimal fibroplasia, the proliferation of myofibroblasts of the intimal layer of the vessels, can also be observed. This lesion is responsible for luminal narrowing at the site of the afferent arteriole, which culminates in glomerular ischaemia and focal and global glomerulosclerosis. Arteriolar hyalinosis and interstitial fibrosis are non-specific findings observed in patients with chronic kidney disease thought to be attributed to hypertension, although they can be seen in individuals without hypertension as well.

9.2.2 Pathophysiological effect of acute hypertension on the kidneys

Acute and severe elevations in blood pressure can damage the renal vascular bed by surpassing the autoregulatory threshold in the kidney, known as malignant hypertension. This can result in severe vascular hyalinosis. Distinct types of damage that occur in this setting include: (1) proliferative endarteritis in the interlobar arteries attributed to endothelial damage from barotrauma (barotrauma causes smooth muscle endothelial cells to migrate, causing intimal proliferation); (2) necrotizing arteriolitis, which occurs when fibrin and other plasma elements leak into the vessel wall, resulting in vascular necrosis; and (3) necrotizing glomerulitis, which involves necrosis and proliferation of the glomerulus. Thrombotic microangiopathy can also occur, which results in intravascular haemolysis and destruction of the microcirculation by glomerular thrombi.

9.3 Epidemiology of hypertension-mediated organ damage to the kidney in hypertension

9.3.1 Risk factors for kidney damage due to hypertension

Several factors are associated with an elevated risk of kidney target organ damage due to hypertension, including severity of hypertension, prolonged duration of uncontrolled hypertension, masked hypertension, male sex, low socio-economic status, smoking, obesity, diabetes mellitus, pre-existing chronic kidney disease, and primary aldosteronism. Whilst all patients with hypertension should be monitored for renal dysfunction with annual evaluation of serum creatinine (or cystatin C, if available) and electrolytes, patients with these risk factors should be particularly closely monitored, due to their greater risk of hypertension-mediated organ damage, and may benefit from a more detailed assessment of renal function, including evaluation of the urine sediment and quantitative assessment of the urine albumin-to-creatinine ratio (see Section 9.3). Patients with these risk factors may also benefit from more stringent blood pressure control to reduce the risk of kidney and other hypertension-mediated organ damage (see Sections 9.4. and 9.5). Of note, many of the risk factors for renal dysfunction due to hypertension are also associated with an increased risk of developing hypertension and difficult-to-control (i.e. resistant or refractory) hypertension, further warranting close monitoring of these patients.

9.3.2 Epidemiological evidence of development and progression of chronic kidney disease due to hypertension

There is ongoing debate as to whether hypertension can be the sole aetiological factor responsible for the development of chronic kidney disease. Several observational studies have demonstrated a temporal relationship between elevated blood pressure and subsequent development of new-onset kidney disease. However, these findings are not consistent across all studies. The reason for this mixed evidence may be due to the long period of time over which elevated blood pressure causes kidney target organ damage; patients would need to be followed up for many years longer than the typical study duration to observe the relationship between elevated blood pressure and incident chronic kidney disease. In contrast, there is strong evidence to support the causal relationship between elevated blood pressure and progression of existing chronic kidney disease.

9.4 Clinical evaluation of hypertension-mediated renal damage

Serum creatinine or cystatin C, urinalysis, and urine albumin-to-creatinine ratio should be assessed in all patients with a new diagnosis of hypertension or with chronically uncontrolled hypertension (Table 9.1). Patients with hypertension should continue to be monitored with annual serum creatinine or cystatin C testing, and those at high risk of kidney target organ damage (see Section 9.2.1) may benefit from closer monitoring (e.g. every 3–6 months) and repeat urine testing.

Patients with evidence of hypertension-mediated renal dysfunction disproportionate to their degree of blood pressure control in the office should undergo 24-hour ambulatory blood pressure monitoring to assess for masked hypertension (i.e. normal blood pressures in the office, with elevated blood pressures at home). These patients should also be evaluated for secondary causes of hypertension that can also result in renal dysfunction, independent of the degree of blood pressure control, including primary aldosteronism (by initially checking plasma renin and aldosterone levels) and renal artery stenosis.

9.5 Interventions to reduce the risk of hypertension-mediated kidney dysfunction

Although randomized controlled trial evidence has not demonstrated a benefit from stringent blood pressure control with regard to new-onset renal dysfunction, consistent blood pressure control remains the mainstay of treatment to minimize the risk of hypertension-mediated kidney damage. Most patients with a known diagnosis of hypertension, or without a diagnosis of hypertension whose blood pressures are within 10 mmHg of their goal blood pressure, should undergo out-of-office blood pressure monitoring (24-hour ambulatory blood pressure monitoring or self-monitoring of blood pressure at home). Out-of-office blood pressure monitoring is particularly helpful to monitor for masked hypertension (normal blood pressures in the office, with elevated blood pressures at home) or sustained hypertension (elevated blood pressures both at home and in the office, which sometimes occurs due to transition from, or is mistaken for, white coat hypertension, i.e. isolated office hypertension), and is more closely linked to target organ damage and long-term adverse kidney and cardiovascular outcomes than in-office blood pressure. Optimization of risk factors for hypertension and chronic kidney disease can have synergistic effects on blood pressure control and renal function, such as improved diet and exercise, weight loss in overweight and obese individuals, management of dyslipidaemia, smoking cessation, and glycaemic control in patients with diabetes mellitus.

9.6 Interventions to reduce progression of pre-existing hypertension-mediated kidney damage

For patients who already have chronic kidney disease, there is strong evidence to support stringent blood pressure control for secondary prevention of further target organ damage. Patients also benefit from optimization of other modifiable risk factors for inadequate blood pressure control and chronic kidney disease progression, described in Section 9.4.

Targeted selection of antihypertensive medications can also reduce progression of chronic kidney disease by reducing glomerular hyperfiltration. In patients with known proteinuria, renin–angiotensin-aldosterone system (RAAS) blockade with angiotensin-converting enzyme inhibitors or angiotensin receptor blockers reduces the risk of chronic kidney disease progression. Mineralocorticoid receptor antagonists likely also have antiproteinuric benefits due to their aldosterone-blocking effects, as aldosterone is thought to cause podocyte damage, mesangial proliferation, and proteinuria. In those who cannot tolerate RAAS blockade (e.g. due to medication intolerance, allergy, or hyperkalaemia), non-dihydropyridine calcium channel blockers also have potential antiproteinuric benefits, although their effect on long-term outcomes have not been studied. Dihydropyridine calcium channel blockers, which are more commonly prescribed for management of hypertension than non-dihydropyridine calcium channel blockers due to greater antihypertensive potency, have not been shown to have the same antiproteinuric benefit.

Recent studies have shown that addition of sodium–glucose co-transporter-2 inhibitors to RAAS blockade helps to further slow the progression of chronic kidney disease. These medications block the sodium–glucose co-transporter-2 in the proximal tubule, promoting increased natriuresis. Although RAAS blockade remains the mainstay therapy for managing hypertension in patients with chronic kidney disease and diabetes, sodium–glucose co-transporter-2 inhibitors can be considered as adjunctive therapy and may be a suitable substitute for RAAS blockade if the latter is not tolerated or contraindicated.

9.7 Conclusion

In summary, the kidneys have a 'cause–effect' relationship with hypertension, wherein chronic kidney disease is known to cause hypertension, whilst at the same time, hypertension has been implicated in the aetiology and progression of chronic kidney disease. Strict control of blood pressure has been shown to slow down the progression of renal dysfunction in patients with chronic kidney disease. Patients with hypertension need regular monitoring of their renal function.

KEY REFERENCES

Anderson AH, Yang W, Townsend RR, et al. (2015). Time-updated systolic blood pressure and the progression of chronic kidney disease: a cohort study. Ann Intern Med 162:258–65.

Cushman WC, Evans GW, Byington RP, et al.; ACCORD Study Group (2010). Effects of intensive blood-pressure control in type 2 diabetes mellitus. N Engl J Med 362:1575–85.

Fogo A, Breyer JA, Smith MC, et al. (1997). Accuracy of the diagnosis of hypertensive nephrosclerosis in African Americans: a report from the African American Study of Kidney Disease (AASK) Trial. AASK Pilot Study Investigators. Kidney Int 51:244–52.

Hall JE, Hall ME. Guyton and Hall Textbook of Medical Physiology, 14th edition. London: WB Saunders, 2020.

Huang M, Matsushita K, Sang Y, Ballew SH, Astor BC, Coresh J (2015). Association of kidney function and albuminuria with prevalent and incident hypertension: the Atherosclerosis Risk in Communities (ARIC) study. Am J Kidney Dis 65:58–66.

Jafar TH, Stark PC, Schmid CH, et al. (2003). Progression of chronic kidney disease: the role of blood pressure control, proteinuria, and angiotensin-converting enzyme inhibition: a patient-level meta-analysis. Ann Intern Med 139:244–52.

Perkovic V, Jardine MJ, Neal B, et al. (2019). Canagliflozin and renal outcomes in type 2 diabetes and nephropathy. N Engl J Med **380**:2295–306.

Rahman M, Wang X, Bundy JD, et al. (2020). Prognostic significance of ambulatory BP monitoring in CKD: a report from the Chronic Renal Insufficiency Cohort (CRIC) Study. J Am Soc Nephrol **31**:2609–21.

Wright JT Jr, Bakris G, Greene T, et al. (2002). Effect of blood pressure lowering and antihypertensive drug class on progression of hypertensive kidney disease: results from the AASK trial. JAMA **288**:2421–31.

Wright JT Jr, Williamson JD, Whelton PK, et al.; SPRINT Research Group (2015). A randomized trial of intensive versus standard blood-pressure control. N Engl J Med **373**:2103–16.

CHAPTER 10

The eye in hypertension

Peck Lin Lip

KEY POINTS

- Hypertensive retinopathy is a manifestation of retinal microvascular damage in the eye related to the chronic insult of high blood pressure.
- Classifications of hypertensive retinopathy are simplified to correlate more closely with risk stratification of end-organ damage and prognosis.
- Recent advancements in fundoscopy and digital fundus imaging allows improved and reliable detection of such retinal changes, hence assisting early diagnosis and management of various commonly encountered hypertension-related ocular complications.
- Malignant hypertension needs to be recognized as a medical emergency, although patients classically first present to eye casualty with headache and varied visual complaints.

10.1 Introduction

Hypertensive retinopathy is a manifestation of retinal microvascular damage in the eye related to the chronic insult of high blood pressure. Recent advancements in fundoscopy and digital fundus imaging allow improved and reliable detection of such retinal changes, hence assisting early diagnosis and management of ocular complications. We describe the effects of hypertension on the eye, specifically on the retina, choroid, and optic nerve as separate entities, as each relates to varied visual presentations, management options, and prognoses.

10.2 Pathology and clinical features of hypertensive retinopathy

Ocular circulation has a unique haemodynamic physiology; in particular, the retinal arterioles have independent autoregulation and a specific blood–retina barrier, differing from the underlying choroidal circulation. Chronic hypertension results in: (1) retinal vascular changes (retinal arteriole vasoconstrictive and sclerotic phases); and (2) extravascular retinal changes (retinal haemorrhages and exudative phases), although both often coexist. Increased luminal pressure from hypertension stimulates autoregulation, resulting in vasoconstriction of the retinal arterioles, which subsequently become sclerotic as a permanent chronic change.

The intimal thickening further worsens arteriolar attenuation (arteriovenous (AV) nipping, copper and silver wiring) and endothelial wall damage. Retinal vascular congestion and tortuosity are common late consequences distal to focal arteriolar constriction and AV nipping, predisposing to the development of retinal vein occlusion (RVO).

10.3 Hypertensive retinopathy

Many of the retinal vascular changes may go unnoticed until the extravascular changes are established and involve the macula area, threatening or affecting normal fovea function. The extravascular changes are a result of the blood–retina barrier disturbance/damage, leading to leakage of plasma (retinal oedema and exudate). Star exudate is a descriptive term for lipid exudation deposited in the outer plexiform of Henle's layer in the macular region.

Retinal haemorrhages develop from necrotic vessels bleeding into the nerve fibre layer (flame haemorrhage, a classic diagnostic hypertensive sign) or the inner retinal layer (dot and blot haemorrhages). Cotton-wool spots indicate the next severity of nerve fibre ischaemia from fibrinous necrosis, causing decreased axoplasmic flow and nerve swelling. Similar clinical features of optic nerve swelling, haemorrhages, exudates, and cotton-wool spots would occur around the optic nerve if the destruction happens to arterioles supplying the optic nerve head. Bilateral involvement is termed malignant hypertension, with corresponding high diastolic blood pressure recordings of >130 mmHg. Unilateral optic nerve swelling is termed anterior optic neuropathy, which is also a medical emergency and requires urgent exclusion of inflammatory causes such as giant cell arteritis.

10.4 Hypertensive choroidopathy

Histopathologically, this is focal fibrinoid necrosis of choroidal arterioles leading to infarction of choriocapillaries, resulting in damage of the corresponding retinal pigment epithelium. In the acute phase, these changes may be visible as small yellowish spots, with localized serous retinal detachment (leaking fluorescein dye at the end of fundus fluorescein angiography), termed as Elschnig's spots. When these spots heal, a scar develops and a pigment spot is left surrounded by a depigmented pale halo. Siegrist streaks are linear hyperpigmented streaks seen over damaged choriocapillaries and occur as a result of chronic hypertensive choroidopathy. These choroidal changes often go undetected, as they cause no visual problem.

10.5 Classifications of hypertensive retinopathy

Early classifications of hypertensive retinopathy (Scheie, Keith–Wagener–Barker) provided a comprehensive description of hypertensive retinopathy changes based on direct ophthalmoscopy and corresponded well to pathophysiological changes.

However, the lower grades of these classifications (i.e. grades 1–2) have limited clinical value due to highly subjective variation in differentiating arteriolar changes on direct ophthalmoscopy and their insignificant prognostic impact related to organ damage from hypertension. In addition, grades 3–4 are not progressive stages from grades 1–2. Subsequently, further efforts were made to simplify classifications to correlate more closely with risk stratification of end-organ damage and prognosis. In the 2-tier classification by Dodson *et al.*, 'non-malignant' retinopathy changes indicate generalized cardiovascular risk related to established hypertension; the 'malignant' retinopathy category, however, signifies a significant mortality risk within 2 years if such high-grade hypertension remains untreated. Table 10.1 summarizes the different classifications of hypertensive retinopathy commonly referred to in clinical practice.

10.6 Other changes seen in the eye with hypertension

Hypertension predisposes to many retinovascular diseases such as macroaneurysms, RVO, anterior optic neuropathy, and malignant hypertension which may cause blindness.

10.6.1 Retinal arterial macroaneurysm

Retinal arterial macroaneurysm is a common eye complication, visible as a localized red saccular dilatation of a larger retinal arteriole. Macroaneurysm can occur as a single lesion or multiple lesions, affecting one or both eyes. Although more common in elderly females with weakened arteriolar walls from atherosclerotic and hormonal changes, it can also occur due to elevated hydrostatic pressure from hypertension. This increased pressure leads to further loss of autoregulatory tone and localized arteriolar dilatation. Macroaneurysms may be an incidental finding, causing no visual problem. Its location in the macula and its proximity to the fovea could threaten visual function by causing vascular leakage (Figure 10.1). The indication for treatment depends on its status: (1) active leakage stage (retinal oedema/exudation around a red macroaneurysm); (2) haemorrhage stage (visible as a red globule with surrounding retinal haemorrhage or breakthrough vitreous haemorrhage); and (3) thrombosed stage (visible as a white globule). Both stages 2 and 3 often lead to thrombosis and eventual collapse of the lesion, thereby requiring no further treatment. Focal laser treatment could benefit selected patients with stage 1 disease where exudation involves the macula and threatens vision.

10.6.2 Retinal vein occlusion

RVO is the second most common cause of visual disability due to retinal vascular disease after diabetic retinopathy. RVO has the strongest association with hypertension, as compared to other systemic causes such as diabetes, vasculitis, and blood dyscrasia. Although age is a predisposing factor for atherosclerotic compression on the already damaged and weakened vascular wall, RVO happens

Table 10.1 Classifications of hypertensive retinopathy

Classifications	Scheie (1953)	Keith–Wagener–Barker (1974)	Dodson et al. (1996)	Wong and Mitchell (2004)
Classification basis	Arteriolar and retinal changes		Cardiovascular risk/prognostic indicator	
Stage/grade 1	Widening of arteriole reflex, minimal arteriolar narrowing	General retinal arteriolar narrowing	Non-malignant: generalized arteriolar narrowing, focal constriction (not AV nipping)	Mild: generalized arteriolar narrowing, focal arteriolar narrowing, AV nipping, copper wiring
Stage/grade 2	Definite arteriolar narrowing, focal irregularities + AV nipping	Focal arteriolar narrowing + AV nipping		Moderate: retinal haemorrhages, microaneurysms, CWS, exudates
Stage/grade 3	Copper wire appearance of arterioles, retinal haemorrhages, exudates, CWS, retinal oedema	Presence of flame-shaped retinal haemorrhages, exudates, and CWS	Malignant: retinal haemorrhages, exudates, CWS ± papilloedema	Malignant: moderate retinopathy as above + papilloedema
Stage/grade 4	Silver wiring appearance of arterioles, papilloedema (+ the above)	Papilloedema (+ the above)		

AV, arteriovenous; CWS, cotton-wool spots; papilloedema, bilateral optic disc swelling.

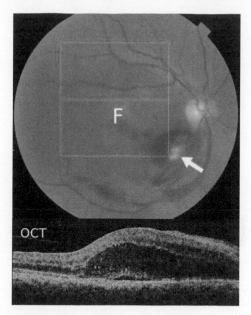

Figure 10.1 Macroaneurysm. A macroaneurysm (arrow) is observed inferior to the optic disc, in proximity to the fovea (F), causing significant retinal oedema, as shown on the retinal cross-sectional optical coherence tomography (OCT) scan. The white centre of the macroaneurysm indicates that thrombosis has occurred within its saccular body, and hence is unlikely to undergo further damage.

commonly when there is an internal retinal venous obstruction (thrombus formation) which may involve the main central vein, or hemispheric (superior or inferior half of the retina) or branch retinal vein territories (Figure 10.2). The two main complications of RVO are macular oedema and retinal ischaemia, with the latter potentially leading to iris and retinal neovascularization, and ultimately late blindness. Currently available treatment options are a series of intravitreal injections of anti-vascular endothelial growth factor, either alone or, in high-risk cases, combined with retinal laser photocoagulation for a permanent effect on the established retinal neovascularization. For patients with existing retinovascular changes, the recommended blood pressure is below 130/80 mmHg.

10.6.3 Malignant hypertension

This is a medical emergency, classically affecting the younger age groups and presenting to the emergency department with headache and varying degrees of visual disturbance. Diagnosis is made when there are bilateral peripapillary retinal haemorrhages, exudates/retinal oedema, with or without optic disc swelling, and

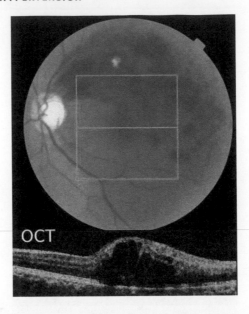

Figure 10.2 Branch retinal vein occlusion. A branch retinal vein occlusion presents as classic flame haemorrhages along the obstructed superotemporal vein, with multiple large and small cotton-wool spots indicating ischaemia of the affected area. Vision is affected as retinal oedema has accumulated in the fovea, as shown on the optical computed tomography (OCT) scan.

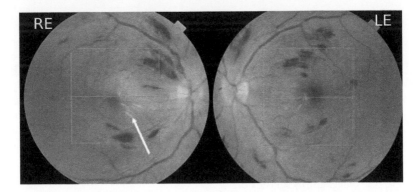

Figure 10.3 Malignant hypertension. Images of a patient 2 weeks after presenting with malignant hypertension. Following normalization of blood pressure, the fundus photos show resolution of papilloedema and improved retinal haemorrhages with residual half star exudate (arrow).

very high blood pressure elevations (often diastolic >130 mmHg). Prompt control of blood pressure is essential here. Retinal changes are reversible within weeks and normalized within months, with no permanent visual damage once the blood pressure is controlled and maintained at normal levels (Figure 10.3). This condition is discussed in detail in Chapter 21.

KEY REFERENCES

Horner F, Lip PL, Mushtaq B, Chavan R, Mohammed B, Mitra A (2020). Combination therapy for macular oedema in retinal vein occlusions: 3-year results from a real-world clinical practice. *Clin Ophthalmol* **14**:955–65.

Lip PL, Cikatricis P, Sarmad A, et al. (2018). Efficacy and timing of adjunctive therapy in the anti-VEGF treatment regimen for macular oedema in retinal vein occlusion: 12-month real-world result. *Eye* **32**:537–45.

Panton RW, Goldberg MF, Farber MD (1990). Retinal arterial macroaneurysms: risk factors and natural history. *Br J Ophthalmol* **74**:595–600.

Shantsila A, Shantsila E, Beevers DG, Lip GYH (2017). Predictors of 5-year outcomes in malignant phase hypertension: the West Birmingham Malignant Hypertension Registry. *J Hypertens* **35**:2310–14.

The Royal College of Ophthalmologists (2022). Retinal vein occlusion (RVO) guidelines 2022 (Feb). Available from: https://www.rcophth.ac.uk/resources-listing/retinal-vein-occlusion-rvo-guidelines/

Wong TY, Mitchell P (2004). Hypertensive retinopathy. *N Engl J Med* **351**:2310–17.

Part 3
Management of hypertension

CHAPTER 11

Overview of guidelines on management of hypertension

Gregory Y. H. Lip and Sunil K. Nadar

KEY POINTS

* American guidelines classify a blood pressure of >130/80 mmHg as hypertension, whilst European and other guidelines have a higher threshold of 140/90 mmHg for diagnosis.
* Different classes of antihypertensive agents are recommended, depending on comorbidities and risk factors.
* Treatment is holistic and should encompass cardiovascular risk management, in addition to blood pressure management
* Latest guidelines recommend a unified blood pressure treatment target, irrespective of comorbidities.

11.1 Introduction

Given the rapid advances in management of patients with hypertension, guidelines on appropriate investigations and treatments (both pharmacological and non-pharmacological) have regularly been issued and updated by learnt bodies to inform the medical community on the optimal approach to such patients.

Many countries issue their own guidelines. However, the major guidelines that are accepted worldwide for clinical use are the joint American guidelines from the American College of Cardiology (ACC) and the American Heart Association (AHA), and the joint European guidelines from the European Society of Hypertension (ESH) and the European Society of Cardiology (ESC). The International Society of Hypertension (ISH) has also recently issued guidelines that can be followed worldwide, especially in countries with limited resources. Guidelines issued by the National Institute for Health and Care Excellence (NICE) in the UK are based on cost-effectiveness and endorsed by the British and Irish Hypertension Society (BIHS).

All the latest guidelines place huge emphasis on overall cardiovascular risk assessment and management, as hypertension is no longer considered a disease in isolation, but as part of a cardiovascular risk continuum. The guidelines issue guidance on measurement of blood pressure (BP), assessment of cardiovascular risk, and investigation of a newly diagnosed hypertensive patient. The guideline documents also give guidance on non-pharmacological and pharmacological treatment and management of special conditions such as hypertension in pregnancy, malignant hypertension, and renal damage. The areas covered in the guideline documents have been covered in other chapters of this book. Here we will concentrate on the treatment algorithms that have been recommended in various guidelines.

11.2 American Heart Association/American College of Cardiology Task Force guidelines on management of hypertension (2017)

The ACC/AHA guidelines on management of hypertension caused a major stir when they were released in 2017. In a major change, as compared to previous guidelines, they lower the threshold for diagnosis of hypertension. They classify a BP of >130/80 mmHg as hypertension, with readings below 120/80 mmHg as normal. Readings in between these are classified as 'high-normal'. These guidelines were based quite strongly on results of the Systolic Blood Pressure Intervention Trial (SPRINT) where most of the BP measurements were from unattended home readings or ambulatory BP readings. Table 11.1 shows the comparison between office readings and corresponding ambulatory home recordings.

Despite the lowered diagnostic threshold, drug therapy is indicated only when the BP is above 140/90 mmHg. For BPs in the range between 130/80 and 140/90 mmHg, drug therapy is indicated only if the global 10-year atherosclerotic cardiovascular disease (ASCVD) risk is >10%.

The change in diagnostic thresholds has huge implications, with the ACC itself acknowledging that this change in threshold would result in an extra 15 million American adults being diagnosed with hypertension. The guidelines place great emphasis on overall cardiovascular risk assessment and risk reduction. There is emphasis on non-pharmacological lifestyle changes.

Table 11.1 Comparison of office, ambulatory, and home blood pressure readings

Clinic blood pressure readings (mmHg)	Home blood pressure readings (mmHg)	Daytime average ambulatory blood pressure reading (mmHg)	Night-time average ambulatory blood pressure reading (mmHg)	24-hour average ambulatory blood pressure reading (mmHg)
120/80	120/80	120/80	100/65	115/75
130/80	130/80	130/80	110/65	125/75
140/90	135/85	135/85	120/70	130/80
160/100	145/90	145/90	140/85	145/90

Table 11.2 Compelling and possible indications for major drug classes

	Compelling indications	Possible indications
Thiazide/ thiazide-like diuretics	Elderly, heart failure, isolated systolic hypertension	
Calcium channel blockers	Elderly, isolated systolic hypertension	Elderly, ischaemic heart disease (rate-limiting non-dihydropyridine agents)
Beta blockers	Ischaemic heart disease	Heart failure (with caution, under supervision)
ACE inhibitors	Heart failure, post-myocardial infarction, type 1 diabetic nephropathy, stroke prevention	Chronic renal disease, type 2 diabetic nephropathy, proteinuric renal disease
Angiotensin receptor blockers	ACE inhibitor intolerance, type 2 diabetic nephropathy, presence of left ventricular hypertrophy	Left ventricular dysfunction post-myocardial infarction
Alpha blockers	Benign prostatic hypertrophy	

ACE, angiotensin-converting enzyme.

In contrast to previous guidelines, the threshold for treatment and the treatment goals have largely been unified for the different patient groups. Apart from patients with low 10-year ASCVD risk of <10% where the treatment threshold is >140/80 mmHg, the treatment threshold for all other groups is a BP of >130/80 mmHg. The treatment goal for all patient groups, including the low cardiovascular risk group, the high cardiovascular risk group, diabetics, and those with pre-existing cardiovascular disease, is <130/80 mmHg. This common treatment goal makes it easier to remember for the treating physician.

The guidelines recommend using any of thiazide diuretics, angiotensin-converting enzyme (ACE) inhibitors, calcium channel blockers, or angiotensin receptor blockers (ARBs) as first-line therapy, along with lifestyle modifications, as these agents have been shown to improve cardiovascular outcomes in clinical trials. Other agents may be used as second-line therapy or in combination with these first-line drugs if there is an insufficient response. In special circumstances, other agents may be considered, based on the clinical condition. These are summarized in Table 11.2. The treatment algorithm is summarized in Figure 11.1.

11.3 Joint European Society of Cardiology/European Society of Hypertension guidelines (2018)

With the release of the slightly controversial American guidelines, it was highly anticipated that the European societies would publish recommendations soon

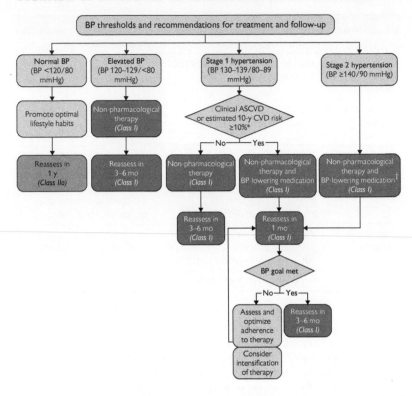

Figure 11.1 Treatment algorithm as suggested by the American College of Cardiology/ American Heart Association hypertension guidelines.

BP, blood pressure; ASCVD, atherosclerotic cardiovascular disease; CVD, cardiovascular disease.

*Using the ACC/AHA Pooled Cohort Equations.

†Consider initiation of pharmacological therapy for stage 2 hypertension with 2 antihypertensive agents of different classes. Patients with stage 2 hypertension and BP$160/100 mm Hg should be promptly treated, carefully monitored, and subject to upward medication dose adjustment as necessary to control BP.

after. They indeed did a year later, with the recommendations fairly unchanged from their 2013 guidance. They kept the definition of hypertension unchanged, with a threshold BP of >140/90 mmHg for the diagnosis of hypertension. The threshold for treatment is also a BP >140/90 mmHg for all groups of patients, irrespective of comorbidities, apart from those aged 80 years and above in whom the threshold is >160/90 mmHg. The treatment goal is first to bring the BP lower than 140/90 mmHg and if tolerated, the ultimate aim is a BP of <130/80 mmHg in most patients. In those aged <65 years, the target is a BP in the range of 120–129/80 mmHg, and in those aged >65 years, the target is a BP in the range of

130–139/80 mmHg. This is irrespective of the cardiovascular risk or the presence or absence of established cardiovascular disease. They specify the reason for giving a treatment target range as they mention that studies have demonstrated harm, rather than benefit, when the BP is lowered to <120/80 mmHg, especially in patients aged >65 years with multiple comorbidities.

Like the American guidelines, the European guidelines also place a lot of emphasis on the role of ambulatory and home BP measurements in the diagnosis and follow-up of patients with hypertension and their use in the diagnosis of masked and white coat hypertension. The guidelines also emphasize the importance of assessing cardiovascular risk in these patients, along with identifying the presence of hypertension-mediated organ damage.

These guidelines also highlight the importance of lifestyle modifications in the management of patients with hypertension and continuation of these efforts even after initiation of pharmacological therapy. The decision to start treatment is summarized in Figure 11.2. As with the American guidelines, they suggest that any of the approved agents (ACE inhibitors, ARBs, calcium channel blockers, diuretics, or beta blockers) can be initiated based on comorbidities. Beta blockers have been included in first-line therapy, especially in special circumstances such as in the presence of ischaemic heart disease, symptomatic angina, or heart failure with reduced ejection fraction, and as an alternative to ACE inhibitors in younger women planning pregnancy.

Once drug therapy has been initiated, in a departure from the previous guidelines, they recommend addition of a second antihypertensive agent early, rather than waiting to achieve the maximal dose of the first agent. Most combinations are encouraged, with the exception of ACE inhibitors with ARBs and beta blockers with thiazide-like diuretics, as the latter combination has been shown to increase the incidence of diabetes. Common combinations that have been shown to be effective are an ACE inhibitor or ARB with a calcium channel blocker or diuretic. They also suggest that many newly diagnosed patients might require initiation with combination therapy and recommend starting with a low-dose combination of two agents, rather than a single agent. In order to improve adherence to medications, they suggest the use of single-pill combination therapy. The special circumstances for use of different agents and the contraindications are similar to the American guidelines and are summarized in Table 11.2.

11.4 British Irish Hypertension Society/NICE guidelines (2019)

NICE and the BIHS updated their guidance on treatment and management of hypertension in 2019. As with other guidelines, they place emphasis on the correct technique for the measurement of BP. They also emphasize the role of ambulatory BP monitoring and home BP readings in the diagnosis and follow-up of patients with hypertension.

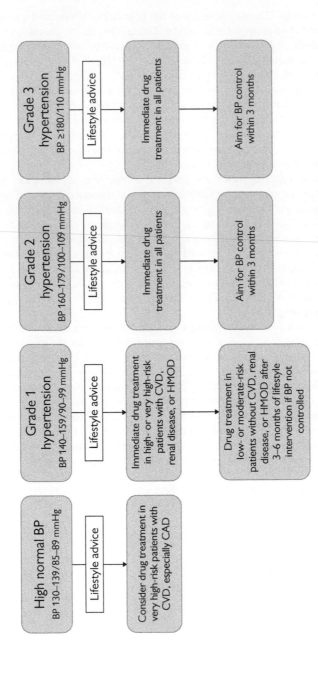

Figure 11.2 Treatment algorithm as recommended by the European Society of Cardiology/European Society of Hypertension guidelines (2018).

BP, blood pressure; CVD, cardiovascular disease; CAD, coronary artery disease; HMOD, hypertension-mediated organ damage.

For the diagnostic threshold, the NICE guidance recommends a cut-off value of 140/90 mmHg for office readings and a daytime value of 135/85 mmHg for ambulatory BP monitoring or home monitoring. The treatment goals are slightly higher than those of the European guidelines, with a target office BP of 140/90 mmHg in those aged 80 and below and a target of 150/90 mmHg as for those above the age of 80. The corresponding values for ambulatory readings, for the groups above are 135/85 mmHg and 145/85 mmHg, respectively.

In contrast to the European guidelines, the British guidelines suggest a step-wise approach of initial monotherapy which is increased before adding the next drug. This is fairly unchanged from their guidance issued in 2011. In brief, step 1 is monotherapy with either an ACE inhibitor or an ARB for patients with low renin states such as young patients or non-Afro-Caribbean patients. For older patients or patients of Afro-Caribbean origin, a calcium channel blocker is recommended. For patients who are unable to tolerate a calcium channel blocker due to oedema or if there are heart failure-like symptoms, a thiazide-like diuretic (chlorthalidone or indapamide) can be started, rather than the conventional thiazide diuretic.

Step 2 would be adding a second drug, for example, an ACE inhibitor to either the calcium channel blocker or the diuretic. The combination of an ACE inhibitor and an ARB should be avoided. Step 3 would be adding all three, and step 4 would be adding a different agent such as a beta blocker, an alpha blocker, or another diuretic. At this stage, it is recommended to refer to a specialist if the BP remains uncontrolled.

Besides pharmacotherapy, the importance of lifestyle changes and adherence to medications is also highlighted. Lowering the overall cardiovascular risk by use of statins and antiplatelet agents (aspirin) is recommended in patients with existing cardiovascular disease and those at high risk of future cardiovascular disease.

11.5 International Society of Hypertension Global Hypertension Practice Guidelines (2020)

These guidelines were developed by the ISH Guidelines Committee, as it was noted that most low- and middle-income countries do not have their own guidelines and often follow those issued by high-income and high-resource countries. And when they do have their own guidelines, they are usually based on guidelines of high-income countries. Implementation of these guidelines may not always be practical due to lack of resources, including lack of trained healthcare professionals, unreliable power supply in rural clinics, poor access to basic office BP devices, limited ability to conduct basic recommended diagnostic procedures, and poor access to affordable, high-quality medications. These guidelines were therefore developed to be used globally, be fit for application in low- and middle-resource countries, and be concise, simple, and easy to use.

To be applicable to all resource settings, they have given optimal standards and essential standards. Optimal standards refer to ideal standards that practitioners should aim to achieve. However, they are aware that resources may not always allow for this and hence have also mentioned essential standards which are the bare minimum that should be achieved.

Diagnosis of hypertension is made when office BP readings are >140/90 mmHg, with a reading of <130/80 mmHg considered normal and readings in the range of 130/80 mmHg to 139/89 mmHg considered to be 'high-normal'. For 24-hour ambulatory BP readings, an average of >130/80 mmHg is considered to be hypertension. These are similar to the European and British guidelines. The threshold to treat, however, is higher than in the other guidelines. In patients with established cardiovascular disease, end-organ damage, or high cardiovascular risk, treatment should be initiated at a BP of >140/90 mmHg. In other low-risk patients, the threshold for treatment is >160/90 mmHg. The target BP goals are also similar to those in the European guidelines, with an optimal target BP of 120–130/70–80 mmHg in all patients aged <65 years or a target BP of 140/90 mmHg in those aged >65 years. The bare minimum 'essential' standard is to lower the BP by at least 20/10 mmHg or achieve a target of <140/90 mmHg in all patients. This control should be achieved within 3 months.

With regard to initiation of pharmacological therapy, the essential standard is to start on any drug that is available or affordable that can lower the BP. The optimal standards, however, are fairly similar to those in the European guidelines and suggest starting with a single-pill combination drug or a two-drug low-dose combination as first line. The first-line combination is ideally that of an ACE inhibitor, or an ARB, with a calcium channel blocker. The next step would be to increase the dose of this combination, with the third step being the addition of a diuretic. The fourth step is the addition of other agents such as spironolactone, beta blockers, alpha blockers, etc., as tolerated.

These guidelines also stress the importance of assessing and lowering cardiovascular risk, the importance of non-pharmacological lifestyle changes, and the importance of adherence to medications. Adapting newer ways to improve adherence and making medications more affordable are important in all countries, and more so in low- and middle-income countries.

11.6 Conclusion

Apart from the difference in the diagnostic cut-off value for hypertension in the American guidelines, most of the major guidelines are fairly similar in their approach to a patient with hypertension. Table 11.3 shows a comparison of the main points of the different guidelines. Removing the different treatment goals and thresholds for different groups of patients has made the guidelines easier and more practical to use. All the guidelines highlight the need for overall cardiovascular risk reduction in patients with hypertension and the importance of adherence to medications and lifestyle changes.

Table 11.3 Comparison of different guidelines

	ACC/AHA 2017	ESC/ESH 2018	NICE/BIHS 2019	ISH-Global 2020
Diagnosis/classification*				
Optimal	–	<120/80	–	–
Normal	<120/80	120–129/80–84	<130/80	<130/85
Elevated/high normal	120–129/80	130–139/85–89	130–139/85–89	130–139/80–89
Stage 1/grade 1	130–139/80–89	140–159/90–99	140–159/90–99	140–159/90–99
Stage 2/grade 2	≥140/90	160–179/100–109	160–179/100–109	>160/100
Grade 3	–	≥180/110	>180/110	–
Treatment thresholds				
Established CVD	≥130/80	>140/90	>140/90	140–159/80–89
Presence of HMOD	≥130/80	>140/90	>140/90	140–159/80–89
DM	≥130/80	>140/90	>140/90	140–159/80–89
10-year CVD risk >10%	≥130/80	>140/90	>140/90	140–159/80–89
No CVD and 10-year risk <10%	≥140/90	>140/90	>140/90	>160/90
Age <65 years	No age-specific guidelines	>140/90	>140/90	No age-specific guidelines
Age 65–79 years	No age-specific guidelines	>140/90	>140/90	No age-specific guidelines
Age >80 years	No age-specific guidelines	>160/90	>150/90	No age-specific guidelines
Treatment targets				
Established CVD	<130/80	<140/90 or <130/80 if tolerated	<140/90 (ABPM 135/85)	A reduction of at least 20/10 mmHg, ideally to <140/90 mmHg in all groups

(continued)

Table 11.3 Continued

	ACC/AHA 2017	ESC/ESH 2018	NICE/BIHS 2019	ISH-Global 2020
Presence of HMOD	<130/80	<140/90 or <130/80 if tolerated	<140/90 (ABPM 135/85)	A reduction of at least 20/10 mmHg, ideally to <140/90 mmHg in all groups
DM	<130/80	<140/90 or <130/80 if tolerated	<140/90 (ABPM 135/85)	A reduction of at least 20/10 mmHg, ideally to <140/90 mmHg in all groups
10-year CVD risk >10%	<130/80	<140/90 or <130/80 if tolerated	<140/90 (ABPM 135/85)	A reduction of at least 20/10 mmHg, ideally to <140/90 mmHg in all groups
No CVD and 10-year risk <10%	<130/80	<140/90 or <130/80 if tolerated	<140/90 (ABPM 135/85)	A reduction of at least 20/10 mmHg, ideally to <140/90 mmHg in all groups
Age <65 years	No age-specific guidelines	120–129/80 mmHg	<140/90 (ABPM 135/85)	120–130/70–80
Age >65 years	No age-specific guidelines	130–139/80 mmHg	<140/90 (ABPM 135/85)	<140/90
Age >80 years	No age-specific guidelines	–	<150/90 (ABPM 145/85)	–

* Based on office blood pressure readings.

All values are in millimetres of mercury.

ACC, American College of Cardiology; AHA, American Heart Association; ESC, European Society of Cardiology; ESH, European Hypertension Society; NICE, National Institute for Health and Care Excellence; BIHS, British Irish Hypertension Society; ISH, International Society of Hypertension; CVD, cardiovascular disease; HMOD, hypertension-mediated organ damage; DM, diabetes mellitus; ABPM, ambulatory blood pressure monitoring.

KEY REFERENCES

Goel H, Tayel H, Nadar SK (2019). Aiming higher in hopes to achieve lower: the European Society of Cardiology/European Society of Hypertension versus the American College of Cardiology/American Heart Association guidelines for diagnosis and management of hypertension. *J Hum Hypertens* **33**:635–8.

National Institute for Health and Care Excellence (2019). Hypertension in adults: diagnosis and management. NICE guideline [NG136]. Available from: https://www.nice.org.uk/guidance/ng136

Unger T, Borghi C, Charchar F, *et al.* (2020). International Society of Hypertension Global Hypertension Practice Guidelines. *Hypertension* **75**:1334–57.

Whelton PK, Carey RM, Aronow WS, *et al.* (2018). 2017 CC/AHA/AAPA/ABC/ACPM/AGS/APhA/ASH/ASPC/NMA/PCNA Guideline for the prevention, detection, evaluation, and management of high blood pressure in adults: a report of the American College of Cardiology/American Heart Association Task Force on Clinical Practice Guidelines. *J Am Coll Cardiol* **71**:e127–248.

Williams B, Mancia G, Spiering W, *et al.*; ESC Scientific Document Group (2018). 2018 ESH/ESC Guidelines for the management of arterial hypertension. *Eur Heart J* **39**:3021 104.

CHAPTER 12

Hypertension and cardiovascular risk management

James P. Sheppard and Sunil K. Nadar

KEY POINTS

* The treatment objective of hypertension is to reduce the risk of cardiovascular disease and its complications.
* This ensures patients have increased life expectancy and improved quality of life.
* In those at high risk of cardiovascular disease, treatment should be focused on addressing all risk factors, and not blood pressure alone.

12.1 Introduction

Hypertension is an important risk factor for the development of cardiovascular disease (CVD). Both systolic and diastolic blood pressures bear a relationship to cardiovascular morbidity and mortality. Hypertension is common in adults over the age of 40 years and is associated with a significant proportion of deaths globally every year.

Management of patients with hypertension traditionally focused on a target for measured blood pressure values and a variety of drugs to achieve this. The recognition that the majority of patients with hypertension have other coexisting risk factors has moved the emphasis to comprehensive management of cardiovascular risk. Indeed, in some countries, blood pressure-lowering treatment is now initiated on the basis of cardiovascular risk alone, rather than blood pressure readings themselves.

The aim of cardiovascular risk factor management is to reduce the incidence of fatal and non-fatal cardiovascular and cerebrovascular events. This is a cost-effective strategy which leads to increased life expectancy and better quality of life. This chapter outlines how cardiovascular risk can be measured, how high-risk patients should be defined, and what treatments, besides blood pressure-lowering therapy, are available for those identified as being at risk.

12.2 Defining cardiovascular risk

Hypertension is only one of many factors which contribute to an individual's overall cardiovascular risk. Diabetes, hyperlipidaemia, and obesity are additional risk factors which can be a manifestation of various lifestyle choices such as high-calorie diet, sedentary lifestyle, and smoking. Multiple coexisting risk factors have a compounding effect in increasing the overall risk. To help better understand an individual's risk in the presence of these factors, a number of cardiovascular risk scores have been developed. These include:

1. The World Health Organization/International Society of Hypertension (WHO/ISH) risk prediction charts estimate the 10-year risk of a fatal or non-fatal myocardial infarction or stroke, based on age, sex, blood pressure, smoking status, total blood cholesterol, and presence or absence of diabetes mellitus. They contain a number of charts appropriate to different global areas.

2. The American College of Cardiology/American Heart Association (ACC/AHA) 10-year cardiovascular risk equation includes age, sex, smoking status, race, body mass index, systolic and diastolic blood pressures, ratio of total cholesterol to high-density lipoprotein (HDL) cholesterol, diabetes, and existing treatment of hypertension as predictors of future disease.

3. The European Society of Cardiology (ESC)'s HeartSCORE equation estimates an individual's 10-year risk of myocardial infarction or stroke, based on age, sex, smoking status, systolic blood pressure, and ratio of total cholesterol to HDL cholesterol.

4. The Joint British Societies for the prevention of cardiovascular disease (JBS3) cardiovascular risk equation estimates the lifetime risk of developing coronary heart disease (CHD) and stroke. Factors taken into consideration include age, sex, smoking status, ethnicity, body mass index, family history of premature CHD, social deprivation, systolic blood pressure, ratio of total cholesterol to HDL cholesterol, and pre-existing conditions such as hypertension, rheumatoid arthritis, type 2 diabetes, and chronic kidney disease.

The appropriate score to use will depend on the population from which a patient originates. For example, the ESC's HeartSCORE equation has been recalibrated for different European populations. The JBS3 and ACC/AHA cardiovascular risk equations include predictors specific to ethnic minority groups found in the United Kingdom and United States, respectively. Other cardiovascular risk scores may be more appropriate for those living in other parts of the world.

In contrast to most cardiovascular risk scores, the JBS3 equation estimates an individual's lifetime risk of CVD. This is thought to be useful for younger patients in particular, as a tool to educate individuals about the importance of risk factor control. However, the clinical utility in guiding treatment using this approach has been questioned, since most cardiovascular prevention therapies have only been tested for relatively short periods of follow-up (i.e. the effects over an individual's lifetime are unknown) and studies based entirely on cardiovascular risk have given conflicting results.

Some patients may have pre-existing conditions such as established CVD, familial hypercholesterolaemia, chronic kidney disease, carotid or femoral plaques, or a coronary artery calcium score >100. For these patients, an additional cardiovascular risk assessment may be unnecessary since their risk is high enough to justify treatment on the basis of their condition alone, regardless of the underlying blood pressure (Table 12.1).

12.3 Managing risk factors that affect cardiovascular disease

A number of risk factors for CVD are inherent in an individual and are not modifiable. These include age, male sex, family history, and ethnicity. Pre-existing conditions, such as CVD, diabetes mellitus, and left ventricular hypertrophy, and markers of end-organ damage, such as elevated serum creatinine, microalbuminuria, and reduced estimated glomerular filtration rate (eGFR), also confer an increased risk and cannot be modified.

Modifiable risk factors, such as blood pressure, lipids, blood sugars, and smoking, can be favourably altered by either drug therapy or behavioural change. Those at highest risk should be prioritized with more intensive therapy. Table 12.1 summarizes the European hypertension guidelines on management of cardiovascular risk. Lifestyle interventions are encouraged for all individuals with high-normal blood pressure, regardless of risk factors. In addition, for those with grade 2 or 3 hypertension and high-risk grade 1 hypertension, drug treatment is also recommended. Further treatment of lipids, glycated haemoglobin (HbA1c), and platelets should be considered for patients with specific underlying risk factors. Targeting of therapy at those with the highest risk aims to maximize benefit whilst minimizing the adverse effects.

12.4 Non-drug interventions to reduce cardiovascular risk

Lifestyle modification has a role to play in reducing cardiovascular risk. Many of these interventions can help lower blood pressure or delay progression to conditions such as diabetes. These measures are generally helpful, but not proven, to prevent complications from CVD and compliance in the long term is often poor.

Lifestyle interventions are aimed at the following:

- Reducing intake of total calories, salt, and fat in the daily diet. This helps in a number of ways. Reducing dietary sodium intake (salt) has been shown to reduce blood pressure. Reduced calorie intake allows weight reduction in overweight individuals, which has a beneficial effect on blood pressure.

Table 12.1 ESC/ESH classification of hypertension stages in the presence of risk factors and association with overall risk of cardiovascular disease

Hypertension disease staging	Other risk factors, HMOD, or disease	BP (mmHg) grading			
		High normal SBP 130–139 DBP 85–89	Grade 1 SBP 140–159 DBP 90–99	Grade 2 SBP 160–179 DBP 100–109	Grade 3 SBP ≥180 or DBP ≥110
Stage 1 (uncomplicated)	No other risk factors	Low risk	Low risk	Moderate risk	High risk
	One or two risk factors	Low risk	Moderate risk	Moderate to high risk	High risk
	≥3 risk factors	Low to moderate risk	Moderate to high risk	High risk	High risk
Stage 2 (asymptomatic disease)	HMOD, CKD grade 3, or diabetes mellitus without organ damage	Moderate to high risk	High risk	High risk	High to very high risk
Stage 3 (established disease)	Established CVD, CKD grade ≥4, or diabetes mellitus with organ damage	Very high risk	Very high risk	Very high risk	Very high risk

HMOD, hypertension-mediated organ damage; BP, blood pressure; SBP, systolic blood pressure; DBP, diastolic blood pressure; CKD, chronic kidney disease; CVD, cardiovascular disease.

Reproduced with permission from Williams, B. Mancia G, Spiering W, et al. ESC Scientific Document Group, 2018 ESC/ESH Guidelines for the management of arterial hypertension: The Task Force for the management of arterial hypertension of the European Society of Cardiology (ESC) and the European Society of Hypertension (ESH), European Heart Journal, Volume 39, Issue 33, 01 September 2018, Pages 3021–3104, https://doi.org/10.1093/eurheartj/ehy339.

- Increasing the intake of fruit and vegetables. Increases in daily potassium intake and a diet high in fruit and vegetables have been shown to reduce blood pressure.

- Regular exercise. Regular physical activity reduces blood pressure and body fat. Additional benefits such as improved insulin sensitivity and an increase in HDL cholesterol are also seen. Moving away from a sedentary lifestyle is important in maintaining an ideal body weight.

- Moderation of alcohol consumption. Studies have consistently shown that individuals who consume small or moderate amounts of alcohol have a lower cardiovascular mortality than non-drinkers. Heavy drinking is associated with significant morbidity.

- Smoking causes a rise in blood pressure and heart rate. Smoking cessation may not directly lower blood pressure, but it significantly reduces cardiovascular risk. Smoking cessation should be offered as part of a structured programme, including counselling and nicotine replacement therapy.

12.5 Drug interventions to reduce cardiovascular risk

The decision to treat other risk factors is based on the added risk in each hypertensive individual. Treatment strategies include the following.

12.5.1 Antiplatelet and anticoagulant therapy

The benefits and risks of antithrombotic therapy in hypertensive patients have been examined in a Cochrane review (2011) including four randomized controlled trials and 44,102 patients. Only one trial—the Hypertension Optimal Treatment (HOT) Study—showed a benefit of aspirin treatment in terms of reduction in major cardiovascular events (by 15%) and acute myocardial infarction (by 36%), with no effect on stroke or intracerebral haemorrhage. However, aspirin treatment was associated with a 65% increased risk of major haemorrhagic events. Patients with serum creatinine levels of >115 μmol/L (>1.3 mg/dL) and those with a higher cardiovascular risk at baseline had a favourable risk–benefit balance. No other studies identified in this review found a benefit of aspirin treatment or any other antithrombotic treatment (clopidogrel or warfarin) in hypertensive patients. There were no studies of direct oral anticoagulants in this population. In hypertensives at lower baseline risk, the harm of aspirin was found to be similar to the benefits. Aspirin is therefore not recommended for primary prevention in hypertensive patients without evidence of CVD.

Clinical guidelines from Europe, the United Kingdom, and the United States recommend that patients with pre-existing CVD be considered for long-term treatment with low-dose aspirin (secondary prevention). This is because aspirin significantly reduces the risk of recurrent vascular events in this population, although the risk of extracranial bleeds is almost doubled. Patients who have had previous bleeding problems associated with aspirin should be considered for treatment with clopidogrel. Because of the risk of bleeding with aspirin, the benefits of treatment are only likely to outweigh the harms in patients who have a 15–20% 10-year cardiovascular risk. In such patients, aspirin should only be started once good blood pressure control has been achieved, to minimize the risk of haemorrhagic stroke.

12.5.2 Lipid-lowering agents

Several studies have demonstrated the benefit of statins in lowering cardiovascular events. In the Heart Protection Study, administration of simvastatin to patients with established CVD led to a marked reduction in cardiac and cerebrovascular events, compared to placebo. Treated hypertensives accounted for 41% of the entire cohort and the treatment effect was seen in this subgroup as well, irrespective of the type of antihypertensive agent used. Similar results were obtained with pravastatin in the Pravastatin in Elderly Individuals at Risk of Vascular Disease (PROSPER) study in which 62% of trial subjects were hypertensive. Atorvastatin has also been shown to be effective in preventing CVD in the Anglo-Scandinavian Cardiac Outcomes Trial (ASCOT). Most clinical guidelines therefore recommend statins in patients up to the age of at least 80 years who have established CVD or long-term (at least 10 years) diabetes. In all these patients, the goal for serum total and low-density lipoprotein (LDL) cholesterol should be set at <4.5 mmol/L (175 mg/dL) and <2.5 mmol/L (100 mg/dL), respectively, although lower goals may also be considered, i.e. <4.0 and <2 mmol/L (155 and 80 mg/dL, respectively).

Three trials— the Antihypertensive and Lipid-Lowering Treatment to Prevent Heart Attack Trial (ALLHAT), ASCOT, and the Heart Outcomes Prevention Evaluation-3 (HOPE-3) trial—have evaluated the benefits associated with use of statins (pravastatin, atorvastatin, and rosuvastatin, respectively) specifically among patients with hypertension. Whilst ALLHAT did not demonstrate any benefit with pravastatin in hypertensive patients with CVD, ASCOT demonstrated a substantial benefit to the group that was given atorvastatin. HOPE-3 showed that rosuvastatin reduces the risk of major cardiovascular events in patients with intermediate risk, although subgroup analyses suggested this effect was only present at lower systolic blood pressures (<131.5 mmHg). The contrasting results seen in these trials may be explained by a greater relative difference in total and LDL cholesterol achieved among the actively treated participants versus the control group in those trials showing a benefit.

In light of this evidence, the European Society of Hypertension (ESH) and ESC guidelines on management of hypertension recommend statin therapy in hypertensive patients aged <80 years at high risk of CVD. They also suggest treatment should be considered in those who have low to moderate cardiovascular risk. Target levels for serum total and LDL cholesterol should be the same as those for non-hypertensive patients. For patients who do not reach targets or whose HDL cholesterol or triglyceride levels remain abnormal (e.g. <1.0 mmol/L and

>2.3 mmol/L, respectively), addition of ezetimibe or other therapies, as well as referral to a specialist service, may be indicated.

12.5.3 Control of blood sugars

The aim of management of blood sugars is early detection with the goal to prevent progression to diabetes. Diabetes and impaired glucose tolerance are significant risk factors for the development of CVD. Hypertension is common with type 2 diabetes, and diabetic hypertensive patients have a marked increase in total cardiovascular risk. Similarly, hypertension is associated with an increased risk of developing type 2 diabetes. Strict control of blood sugars is important in these patients. In the UK Prospective Diabetes Study (UKPDS), hypertensive patients with type 2 diabetes benefited from intensive blood glucose control through a reduction in microvascular complications. Other studies have shown protection against macrovascular complications with strict glycaemic control as well.

According to guidelines for management of diabetes, the treatment goals are set at ≤6.0 mmol/L (108 mg/dL) for plasma preprandial glucose concentrations (average of several measurements), and at <6.5% for HbA1c. Treatment of diabetic hypertensive patients is discussed in detail in Chapter 24.

12.6 Conclusion

In conclusion, management of hypertension should not be limited to controlling blood pressure in order to reduce the risk of CVD. Management should include an overall assessment of cardiovascular risk, with treatment of blood pressure, lipids, and blood glucose considered, depending on an individual's underlying risk. Guidelines by the British and Irish, American, and European societies of hypertension all recommend lifestyle modification and treatment with antihypertensives, statins, and (in some cases) antiplatelet agents in order to reduce this risk. Thus, treating a hypertensive individual entails a comprehensive and holistic cardiovascular risk management strategy.

KEY REFERENCES

JBS3 Board (2014). Joint British Societies' consensus recommendations for the prevention of cardiovascular disease (JBS3). *Heart* **100** Suppl 2:ii1–67.

National Institute for Health and Care Excellence (2019). Hypertension in adults: diagnosis and management. NICE guideline [NG136]. Available from: https://www.nice.org.uk/guidance/ng136

Padwal R, Strauss S, McAlister FA, *et al.* (2001). Cardiovascular risk factors and their effects on the decision to treat hypertension: evidence based review. *BMJ* **322**:977–80.

Whelton PK, Carey RM, Aronow WS, *et al.* (2017). ACC/AHA/AAPA/ABC/ACPM/AGS/APhA/ASH/ASPC/NMA/PCNA guideline for the prevention, detection, evaluation, and management of high blood pressure in adults: a report of the American

College of Cardiology/American Heart Association Task Force on Clinical Practice Guidelines. *J Am Coll Cardiol* **71**:2199–269.

Williams B, Mancia G, Spiering W, *et al.* (2018). ESC/ESH Guidelines for the management of arterial hypertension. *Eur Heart J* **39**:3021–104.

World Health Organization. *Prevention of Cardiovascular Disease—Pocket Guidelines for Assessment and Management of Cardiovascular Risk.* Geneva: World Health Organization, 2007.

CHAPTER 12

CHAPTER 13

Non-pharmacological management of hypertension

Benjamin J. R. Buckley and Stephanie J. Finnie

> **KEY POINTS**
>
> * Lifestyle modifications are a first-line therapy for optimal hypertension management.
> * Improvements in lifestyle, including increasing physical activity levels and improving diet, contribute to lowering overall cardiovascular disease risk, in addition to improved blood pressure control.
> * Regular exercise, maintenance of healthy body weight, and adhering to a healthy diet complement pharmacological treatment

13.1 Introduction

The importance of a healthy lifestyle is well understood for primary and secondary prevention of cardiovascular disease. Indeed, a meta-epidemiological study including 16 meta-analyses, with nearly 400,000 participants, found no difference in mortality between exercise and drug interventions in secondary prevention of cardiovascular disease and diabetes.

As the majority of patients with hypertension who take blood pressure medication fail to reach treatment goals, non-pharmacological interventions are an important addition to improve management and clinical outcomes. Numerous randomized controlled trials and real-world, population-based studies have emphasized the importance of lifestyle changes as an integral component of lowering blood pressure in both patients with hypertension and those with prehypertension. Lifestyle modification is therefore the first-line antihypertensive treatment guideline in the management of hypertension. In this chapter, we discuss new evidence and recommendations related to lifestyle modification, including exercise and nutritional components, as important antihypertensive therapies. Despite such guidelines, it has been estimated that nearly a third of the population are insufficiently physically active to maintain good health and prevent non-communicable diseases such as cardiovascular disease, diabetes, and cancer.

13.2 Exercise

The World Health Organization 2020 physical activity guidelines recommend 150–300 minutes of moderate-intensity physical activity or 75–150 minutes of vigorous-intensity physical activity, or a combination of the two, per week. This is in addition to resistance exercise 2 days per week. In treatment and prevention of hypertension, the International Society of Hypertension and the American College of Sports Medicine recommend moderate-intensity aerobic exercise (e.g. walking, jogging, cycling, yoga, or swimming) for 30 minutes 5–7 days per week. Aerobic training should also be supplemented with resistance or strength-based exercise on 2–3 days per week. Patients with uncontrolled severe hypertension (i.e. systolic ≥180 mmHg and/or diastolic ≥110 mmHg), however, should contact their physician before starting an exercise programme.

A 2019 network meta-analysis of 391 randomized controlled trials assessed the effects of exercise and medication on systolic blood pressure. Of these, 197 studies evaluated exercise interventions (10,461 participants) and 194 evaluated antihypertensive medications (29,281 participants). Compared with non-exercise controls, all types of exercise (including combination of endurance and resistance) and all classes of antihypertensive medications were effective in lowering baseline systolic blood pressure. Among hypertensive populations, there were no significant differences in systolic blood pressure-lowering effects of commonly used antihypertensive medications (−8.8 mmHg), when compared to exercise (−9 mmHg), endurance (−8.7 mmHg), dynamic resistance exercise (−7.2 mmHg), or combined exercise (−13.5 mmHg)). However, when including non-hypertensive populations in the analyses, antihypertensive medication was more effective at reducing blood pressure. Therefore, the blood pressure-lowering effects of exercise seem to be more potent in hypertensive patients, which is nevertheless a promising message.

Interestingly, exercise also promotes acute cardioprotective effects. A meta-analysis found that regardless of participant, measurement, and intervention characteristics, a single bout of exercise elicits an acute reduction of 4.8 mmHg in blood pressure. A range of risk factors contribute to hypertension, including atherosclerosis, insulin resistance, dyslipidaemia, upregulated sympathetic drive, and decreased beta cholinergic receptor sensitivity. Centrally, all of these factors can be influenced by regular exercise training, yet unlikely explain the observed acute antihypertensive effects. Moreover, the impact of exercise on traditional cardiovascular risk factors does not fully explain the beneficial effect of exercise on major adverse cardiovascular events and mortality. To this end, the potent antihypertensive effects of regular exercise may, at least in part, be explained by improvement in vascular function. Specifically, regular exercise training is associated with upregulation of endothelium-derived nitric oxide synthase, a potent vasodilator, which is critical to vascular tone.

A combination of endurance and resistance training may be more protective than either modality alone. One explanation is that each modality elicits a cardioprotective effect via different mechanisms. Resistance exercise is often a *forgotten tool* in the promotion of physical activity and exercise training. A recent prospective study, including 72,560 men and 59,764 women who were followed up for 4 years, found an inverse association between skeletal muscle mass and blood pressure, as well as the number of new patients receiving antihypertensive medication. These findings corroborate previous longitudinal evidence, such as the bone health study, which found that skeletal muscle attenuation was a risk factor for incident hypertension. When the sample was categorized into ascending quartiles of skeletal muscle mass, there was a clear dose–response relationship, with increased muscle mass associated with a lower incidence of hypertension in both females and males. Thus, resistance training, which is known to attenuate sarcopenia (and even enhance skeletal muscle mass), is a promising additional therapy for primary and secondary antihypertensive therapy. Skeletal muscle mass may therefore help elucidate the antihypertensive properties of chronic resistance training. Although the precise mechanisms explaining the relationship between muscle mass and hypertension are not yet fully understood, insulin resistance, inflammatory pathways, myokines, and arterial stiffness are likely involved.

Whilst antihypertensive drugs have dominated the hypertensive therapy research arena, their effects are limited to blood pressure, often eliciting negative side effects, and do not affect muscle mass, vascular function, or indeed mental well-being. In contrast, exercise offers a systemic benefit (physical, mental, and potentially social) and enhances vascular function and muscle mass, subsequently contributing to blood pressure-lowering properties at a relatively low cost. Therefore, renewed attention to exercise is warranted as a non-pharmacological strategy to better prevent and manage hypertension via promotion of muscle mass and vascular function.

13.3 Diet and nutrition

A 2016 systematic review and meta-analysis of 24 randomized controlled trials, including nearly 24,000 participants, estimated that the overall effect of dietary interventions on systolic blood pressure was −3.1 mmHg. However, studies evaluating the effect of diet on blood pressure are highly heterogeneous, with differences in duration of interventions, measures of adherence, and participant demographics having a substantial impact on the effect. Indeed, the Dietary Approaches to Stop Hypertension (DASH) diet, which promotes reduction of sodium and inclusion of foods rich in nutrients that may help lower blood pressure, such as potassium, calcium, and magnesium, had the largest effect on systolic blood pressure (−7.6 mmHg). A 2019 Cochrane systematic review and meta-analysis (30 randomized controlled trials; 12,461 participants) investigated the effect of the Mediterranean diet for primary and secondary prevention of cardiovascular disease. They found a mean reduction of 3 mmHg in systolic blood pressure. A diet rich in whole grains, fruits, vegetables, polyunsaturated fats, and dairy products and low in sugar and saturated and trans fats, in accordance with the Mediterranean diet, is recommended by the International Society of Hypertension. Table 13.1 summarizes the quality of evidence for several nutritional components and their ability to reduce blood pressure or prevent hypertension.

Aligned with the notion that the Mediterranean diet is protective against hypertension, a systematic review and meta-analysis of seven trials and 32 observational studies found that a vegetarian diet was associated with a reduction in mean blood pressure, compared to an omnivore diet. Specifically, the seven clinical trials (311 participants) found that a vegetarian diet was associated with an average reduction of 4.8 mmHg (systolic) and 2.2 mmHg (diastolic) blood pressure, whereas the 32 observational studies (21,604 participants) demonstrated an associated reduction of 6.9 and 4.7 mmHg in systolic and diastolic blood pressures, respectively.

Table 13.1 Quality of evidence for nutritional components and the impact on blood pressure reduction

Strong evidence	Some evidence	Not scientifically supported
Mediterranean-style diet	Vitamin C	Potassium
Dietary nitrates	Cocoa flavonoids	Pycnogenol
Reducing dietary salt (sodium)	Proteins, peptides, and amino acids	Taurine
Moderate coffee consumption	Coenzyme Q10	Smoking cessation
Moderate tea consumption	Melatonin	Alcohol reduction
Omega-3 polyunsaturated fatty acids	Aged garlic extract	
Dietary magnesium		
Calcium supplementation		

'Strong evidence' refers to evidence class I or IIa and evidence level A or B. 'Some evidence' refers to evidence class IIa or IIb and evidence level B. 'Not scientifically supported' refers to evidence class III and evidence level C.

Evidence class: class I, evidence and/or general agreement that a given treatment or procedure is beneficial, useful, and effective; class IIa, weight of evidence/opinion is in favour of usefulness/efficacy; class IIb, usefulness/efficacy is less well established by evidence/opinion; class III, evidence or general agreement that the given treatment or procedure is not useful/effective and, in some cases, may be harmful.

Evidence level: level A, data derived from multiple randomized clinical trials or their meta-analysis; level B, data derived from single randomized clinical trial or large, non-randomized studies; level C, consensus or opinion of experts and/or small studies, retrospectives studies, and registries.

In addition to macro-diet recommendations such as the DASH, Mediterranean, and vegetarian diets, individual food groups, and even specific nutrients, may also have a beneficial effect with lowering blood pressure (Table 13.1). For example, increasing the intake of leafy vegetables and beetroot, which are high in nitrates (a potent vasodilator), have been shown in meta-analytic data of placebo-controlled randomized trials to be associated with a dose-dependent reduction in blood pressure (average effect −4.4 mmHg).

The effectiveness of restricting dietary sodium has also been demonstrated in more than one Cochrane systematic review and meta-analysis. Sodium reduction from high-level intake (201 mmol/day) to below the recommended upper level of 100 mmol/day was associated with a reduction in systolic blood pressure of only 1 mmHg in white participants with normotension. However, in white participants with hypertension, this reduction increased to 5.5 mmHg. The effect in black and Asian populations seems to be even greater, although further research is needed. Further, increasing dietary potassium intake may reduce the risk of hypertension, as shown in some observational research, although higher-quality evidence is warranted. Still, the sodium-to-potassium ratio may be more important in prevention of hypertension than manipulating either nutrient in isolation.

The National Institute for Health and Care Excellence (NICE) guidelines for management of hypertension advise health professionals to 'discourage excessive consumption of coffee and other caffeine-rich products'. Experimental studies have shown that caffeine can raise levels of adrenaline, noradrenaline, and cortisol, all of which can lead to an increase in blood pressure. However, recent literature reviews suggest an unpredicted protective effect of habitual coffee consumption towards the occurrence of cardiovascular events. There is currently no general consensus on the effect of caffeine on blood pressure, with the effects of caffeine dependent on several variables such as daily dose, coffee-drinking habits, and patients' pre-existing blood pressure.

A 2018 systematic review and dose–response meta-analysis of ten cohort studies (243,869 participants) reported that the risk of hypertension was reduced by 2% with each cup/day increment of coffee consumption, with up to 10% reduced risk with eight cups/day, relative to non-coffee drinkers. Possible mechanisms include diuretic and natriuretic activity of caffeine—although it is possible it is not caffeine, but other active compounds, either in coffee or associated in diets of those with high coffee intake, that may explain the dose-dependent inverse association between coffee consumption and risk of hypertension. Other ingredients in coffee, such as potassium, magnesium, and antioxidants, may contribute to the beneficial effect. In addition, chlorogenic acid (a polyphenol found in coffee) exhibits anti-inflammatory activity via inhibition of tumour necrosis factor alpha (TNF-α) and interleukin 6 (IL-6) pathways. Further research is required to attempt to determine a causal relationship and rule out the possibility of residual confounding.

A large number of dietary flavonoids have been shown to elicit vascular protection, including antioxidant and anti-inflammatory effects, as well as improve nitric oxide bioavailability and endothelial function. A Cochrane meta-analysis of 40 treatment comparisons (1804 participants) revealed a small, but statistically significant, blood pressure-reducing effect (−1.8 mmHg) of flavanol-rich cocoa products, compared to the control. Subgroup analyses demonstrated larger reductions in hypertensive patients (mean effect −4 mmHg systolic blood pressure).

In addition to the Mediterranean diet, promotion of leafy vegetables, and even following a vegetarian diet, a number of individual food groups and nutrients may have a positive impact on blood pressure, either in isolation or combined with other active ingredients and pharmacology. Thus, diet seems to be a powerful tool for primary and secondary prevention of hypertension. Nevertheless, a number of variables appear to impact the magnitude of blood pressure reduction when investigating the impact of nutrition. These include, but are not limited to, study design and blinding, 'active' versus 'inactive' control groups, study duration, and participant characteristics (age, ethnicity, health status, sex, etc.). Such caveats need to be considered when determining the impact of an intervention, especially something as complex as diet.

13.4 Smoking

Smoking is a considerable risk to public health, responsible for over 6 million deaths worldwide. It is a major risk factor for several diseases, including lung cancer, coronary heart disease, and stroke. NICE guidelines for management of hypertension support smoking cessation, given the broad benefits on cardiovascular risk reduction. However, the specific association between smoking and blood pressure is more complicated.

Epidemiological studies have generally reported lower blood pressures among current smokers, compared to non-smokers. A recent meta-analysis of 141,317 individuals from 23 population-based studies reported current smoking, as compared to never smoking, was associated with lower systolic and diastolic blood pressures (−2.4 and −1.93 mmHg, respectively). Current smoking was even associated with a lower risk of hypertension and severe hypertension. Short-term smoking cessation has been suggested to produce reductions in blood pressure, heart rate, and sympathetic activity. A randomized crossover study investigated the effects of 1-week smoking cessation on blood pressure and heart rate in 39 male normotensive habitual smokers. The 24-hour ambulatory blood pressure was significantly lower in the non-smoking period, compared to the smoking period (by 3.5 mmHg systole and 1.9 mmHg diastole), as was the 24-hour heart rate (by 7.3 beats/minute). However, a 4-year observational follow-up study found that sustained smoking cessation resulted in increased blood pressure and incidence of hypertension. The adjusted relative risks of hypertension in those who had quit smoking for <1, 1–3, and ≥3 years were 0.6 (95% confidence interval (CI) 0.2–1.9), 1.5 (95% CI 0.8–2.8), and 3.5 (95% CI 1.7–7.4), respectively, compared to current smokers.

Various confounding factors could explain this association between smoking cessation and hypertension. For example, weight gain is often reported in those who successfully quit smoking (i.e. smokers tend to have a lower body mass index than non-smokers). However, the previously discussed findings demonstrated similar results among those who lost weight, gained weight, and maintained weight. Thus, data support a short-term reduction in blood pressure, but a longer-term increase for those who stop smoking. The mechanisms for this are deserving of future investigation.

In conclusion, more research is required to elucidate the complex relationship between smoking and blood pressure. Current smokers have been observed to have lower blood pressures than non-smokers, but higher resting heart rates, supporting the notion that smoking may exert its detrimental effects on cardiovascular disease, at least partially, by increasing the resting heart rate. Sustained smoking cessation may counterintuitively result in an increase in blood pressure. However, given current evidence suggests that smoking exerts its negative effects on the cardiovascular system via mechanisms separate to elevated blood pressure, smoking cessation is still one of the best things a smoker can do to improve their health.

13.5 Alcohol

Abuse of alcohol is a major public health problem and one of the biggest avoidable risks of disease and death. It also carries a substantial economic burden, costing the National Health Service (NHS) around £3.5 billion per year. NICE guidelines advise men and women to drink no more than 14 units of alcohol per week, with emphasis on spreading drinking over 3 or more days, and highlight the importance of alcohol-free days. However, the question of what constitutes safe alcohol consumption remains debated.

Epidemiological and clinical studies have demonstrated that chronic alcohol consumption (>3 drinks/day; 30 g ethanol) is associated with an increased incidence of hypertension and an increased risk of cardiovascular diseases. The magnitude of increased blood pressure in heavy drinkers averages approximately 5–10 mmHg. In the Framingham cohort, there was an increase of 7 mmHg in mean arterial pressure when heavy alcohol users were compared to all other subjects. The extensive risks of harmful alcohol intake on other aspects of health also need to be considered.

According to existing evidence, not all levels of alcohol are bad; *the dose makes the poison ... or the therapy.* For example, research suggests that moderate consumption of alcohol can be beneficial to the cardiovascular system and even reduce blood pressure. Moderate drinking is generally considered to be two drinks a day for men aged <65, one drink a day for men aged >65, and one drink a day for women of any age. A drink is 355 mL of beer, 148 mL of wine, or 44 mL of 80-proof distilled spirits. It also seems that reducing alcohol consumption is only beneficial for those who drink an excessive amount. A recent systematic review and meta-analysis including 36 trials with 2865 participants investigated the effect of a reduction in alcohol consumption on blood pressure. In people who drank two or fewer drinks per day, a reduction in alcohol intake was not associated with a significant reduction in blood pressure. However, in people who drank more than two drinks per day, a reduction in alcohol intake was associated with an increased blood pressure reduction. Reduction in systolic blood pressure (−5.50 mmHg) and diastolic blood pressure (−3.97 mmHg) was strongest in participants who drank six or more drinks per day if they reduced their intake by approximately 50%.

Therefore, excessive alcohol is associated with an increased cardiovascular disease risk and an increased incidence of hypertension, particularly for heavy drinkers. Alcohol seems to have a biphasic effect on blood pressure, with a decreased blood pressure up to 12 hours after consumption and an increased blood pressure >13 hours after consumption. This may explain the reduction in blood pressure with regular, but moderate, consumption. Reduction of alcohol consumption seems to be increasingly beneficial for heavier drinkers, thus, heavy drinkers have the most to gain by reducing their alcohol intake.

13.6 Conclusion

Non-pharmacological interventions are an integral part of not only preventing and managing hypertension, but also reducing cardiovascular mortality and morbidity. The importance of physical activity, exercise, and diet needs to be consistently emphasized as powerful primary and secondary preventive tools. Therefore, all treating physicians must allow time with patients to discuss patient goals related to non-pharmacological and lifestyle modifications. Finally, although the biggest effects are seen in the most at-risk patients, it is important to remember the concept: 'an ounce of prevention is worth a pound of cure'.

KEY REFERENCES

Andriani H, Kosasih RI, Putri S, Kuo HW (2020). Effects of changes in smoking status on blood pressure among adult males and females in Indonesia: a 15-year population-based cohort study. BMJ Open 10:e038021.

Cowell OR, Mistry N, Deighton K, et al. (2021). Effects of a Mediterranean diet on blood pressure: a systematic review and meta-analysis of randomized controlled trials and observational studies. J Hypertens 39:729–39.

Graudal NA, Hubeck-Graudal T, Jurgens G (2017). Effects of low sodium diet versus high sodium diet on blood pressure, renin, aldosterone, catecholamines, cholesterol, and triglyceride. Cochrane Database Syst Rev 4:CD004022.

Halperin RO, Gaziano JM, Sesso HD (2008). Smoking and the risk of incident hypertension in middle-aged and older men. Am J Hypertens 21:148–52.

Noone C, Leahy J, Morrissey EC, et al. (2020). Comparative efficacy of exercise and anti-hypertensive pharmacological interventions in reducing blood pressure in people with hypertension: a network meta-analysis. Eur J Prev Cardiol 27:247–55.

Rees K, Takeda A, Martin N, et al. (2019). Mediterranean-style diet for the primary and secondary prevention of cardiovascular disease. Cochrane Database Syst Rev 3:CD009825.

Roerecke M, Kaczorowski J, Tobe SW, Gmel G, Hasan OSM, Rehm J (2017). The effect of a reduction in alcohol consumption on blood pressure: a systematic review and meta-analysis. Lancet Public Health 2:e108–20.

Thuy AB, Blizzard L, Schmidt MD, Luc PH, Granger RH, Dwyer T (2010). The association between smoking and hypertension in a population-based sample of Vietnamese men. J Hypertens 28:245–50.

Unger T, Borghi C, Charchar F, et al. (2020). 2020 International Society of Hypertension Global Hypertension Practice Guidelines. Hypertension 75:1334–57.

Xie C, Cui L, Zhu J, Wang K, Sun N, Sun C (2018). Coffee consumption and risk of hypertension: a systematic review and dose–response meta-analysis of cohort studies. J Hum Hypertens 32:83–93.

Yokoyama Y, Nishimura K, Barnard ND, et al. (2014). Vegetarian diets and blood pressure: a meta-analysis. JAMA Intern Med 174:577–87.

CHAPTER 14

Diuretics in hypertension

Harsh Goel and Ashish Kumar

KEY POINTS

- Diuretics are effective both as sole agents and in combination with other antihypertensive drugs. The choice of agent will depend on various factors, including age, ethnicity, comorbidities, and risk of adverse effects.
- Rigorous monitoring of electrolyte balance and renal function is essential during treatment.
- Loop diuretics are more effective than thiazide diuretics in moderate to advanced chronic kidney disease (glomerular filtration rate <30 mL/min).
- Combination of thiazide or loop diuretics with a potassium-sparing agent may further improve blood pressure control and aid maintenance of normokalaemia.
- Aldosterone antagonists may be especially effective in management of resistant hypertension.

14.1 Introduction

Diuretics have continued to be the cornerstone of antihypertensive therapy for over half a century. In addition, they remain an important component of treatment of heart failure and other hypervolaemic states, including cirrhosis and renal failure. Cost-effectiveness, high compliance, and a proven track record in reducing cardiovascular events and mortality in several randomized controlled trials (RCTs) have made them first-line therapy in many hypertensive patients.

14.2 Classification of diuretics

On the basis of their mechanism and site of action in the nephron (Figure 14.1), diuretics can be broadly classified into three major classes:

- Thiazide diuretics: further subclassified as thiazide (hydrochlorothiazide and bendroflumethiazide) and thiazide-like (indapamide, metolazone, and chlorthalidone)
- Loop-acting diuretics
- Potassium-sparing diuretics: further subdivided into potassium-sparing (triamterene and amiloride) and aldosterone antagonists (spironolactone and eplerenone).

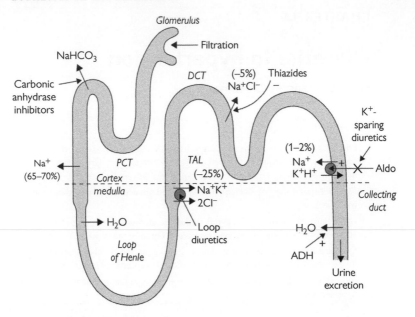

Figure 14.1 Diaphragmatic representation of a nephron, depicting the sites of action of the three major classes of diuretics.

DCT, distal convoluted tubule; PCT, proximal convoluted tubule; Aldo, aldosterone; NaHCO$_3$, sodium bicarbonate; NA, sodium ions; K$^+$, potassium ions; H$_2$O, water; ADH, antidiuretic hormone; Cl, chloride.

14.3 Thiazide diuretics

Thiazides act by blocking the thiazide-sensitive sodium (Na$^+$)/chloride (Cl$^-$) pump in the distal convoluted tubule, preventing sodium and chloride re-absorption, and inducing natriuresis and a negative sodium balance. The resulting reduction in intravascular plasma volume and cardiac output is primarily responsible for the antihypertensive action, although modest vasodilatation of unclear mechanism may play a minor role, especially with longer-acting agents such as chlorthalidone and indapamide. Given the luminal site of action, thiazide efficacy is dependent on proximal tubular organic acid transporter (OAT)-mediated transport to the tubular lumen. Hence, as the glomerular filtration rate (GFR) decreases in chronic kidney disease, accumulating organic acids compete with thiazides for OATs and reduce luminal delivery of the latter, decreasing efficacy. Hence, thiazides are generally not recommended in patients with GFR <30 mL/min.

Although higher doses (≥50 mg of hydrochlorothiazide or equivalent) may produce greater natriuresis, antihypertensive efficacy at these doses is attenuated due to greater activation of the compensatory renin–angiotensin axis. Moreover, most metabolic adverse effects, including hyperglycaemia, hyperuricaemia, and elevated cholesterol level, as well as electrolyte abnormalities, are dose-dependent and represent a significant burden at these doses. A recent systematic review found high-quality evidence that low-dose thiazides as first-line antihypertensives reduced the risk of coronary heart disease (relative risk (RR) 0.72, 95% confidence interval (CI) 0.61–0.84), stroke (RR 0.68, 95% CI 0.60–0.77), cardiovascular events (RR 0.70, 95% CI 0.64–0.76), and mortality (RR 0.89, 95% CI 0.82–0.97). Hence, modern treatment regimens for hypertension have gravitated towards lower dosages (hydrochlorothiazide 12.5–25 mg daily). In this regard, thiazide-like diuretics (chlorthalidone and indapamide) are more potent per milligram than hydrochlorothiazide, hence more effective at lower doses.

14.3.1 Contraindications

- Hypersensitivity to thiazides or sulfonamides
- Uncontrolled gout
- Lithium therapy (bipolar disorder)
- Pregnancy and breastfeeding
- Severe renal impairment.

14.3.2 Adverse effects

The majority of common adverse effects (electrolyte abnormalities, elevated glucose, hyperuricaemia, and elevated cholesterol level) are dose-dependent; hence, low-dose therapy (12.5–25 mg/day of hydrochlorothiazide and chlorthalidone, 1.25 mg/day of indapamide) has become standard of care. Clinically relevant adverse effects include:

- Hypokalaemia (concurrent angiotensin-converting enzyme (ACE) inhibitor may balance this)
- Hyponatraemia (can cause confusion in extreme cases)
- Hypercalcaemia (little clinical significance)
- Hyperuricaemia (avoid or use cautiously in patients with a history of gout, especially when not on urate-lowering therapy)
- Hyperglycaemia (or deterioration in glycaemic control among diabetic patients), in particular with beta adrenergic receptor blockers
- Metabolic alkalosis
- Anorexia, jaundice, pancreatitis, and hepatic coma (should be stopped)
- Leucopenia, agranulocytosis, thrombocytopenia, aplastic anaemia, and haemolytic anaemia

- Orthostatic hypotension (in particular, among the elderly, may necessitate interruption/cessation of therapy)
- Acute interstitial pneumonitis (rare, but potentially life-threatening).

14.3.3 Interactions

A detailed treatise on drug interactions is outside the scope of this text, but care is advised when prescribing thiazide diuretics with oral anticoagulants, steroids, and lithium (lithium toxicity may rapidly develop).

14.3.4 Indications

There has been some discussion for decades regarding the relative efficacy of thiazide versus thiazide-like diuretics. At lower doses recommended in most current guidelines, chlorthalidone (12.5–25 mg/day; ALLHAT, MRFIT, SHEP trials) and indapamide (1.25–2.5 mg/day; HYVET, ADVANCE, and PROGRESS trials) have demonstrated efficacy in reducing cardiovascular events and mortality. On the other hand, evidence regarding hydrochlorothiazide is somewhat mixed (ACCOMPLISH and MRFIT trials). Though there are no head-to-head RCTs comparing thiazide and thiazide-like diuretics, meta-analyses suggest chlorthalidone being superior to hydrochlorothiazide in reducing cardiovascular events and heart failure, even when adjusted for blood pressure reductions by the two agents. Moreover, thiazide-like diuretics, due to a much longer duration of action, likely achieve better 24-hour blood pressure control than shorter-acting thiazides. Hence, many major guidelines, including those from the UK National Institute for Health and Care Excellence (NICE) and the American College of Cardiology/ American Heart Association (ACC/AHA), now recommend chlorthalidone or indapamide over hydrochlorothiazide.

According to the latest NICE recommendations, thiazides are recommended as sole agents in non-diabetic stage 1 hypertensives (or those who have systolic blood pressure <20 mmHg above goal) without advanced renal disease, especially if they are of African or African-Caribbean origin and cannot tolerate a dihydropyridine calcium channel blocker (CCB) (due to oedema). They may be used as first-line agents in patients who have symptoms of heart failure. In addition, thiazides can be combined with either ACE inhibitors (ACEIs) or CCBs (step 2 in NICE guidelines) in case of an inadequate response to one agent. The combination of thiazides with ACEIs is particularly attractive due to physiological synergy, since compensatory renin–angiotensin axis activation induced by the former is blunted by the latter. Finally, thiazides also may be of use in patients with established heart failure or coronary heart disease, as add-on therapy to guideline-based secondary prevention (beta adrenergic blockers, ACEIs), especially in patients with symptoms due to volume overload. Most other guidelines recommend a largely similar approach (ACC/AHA, European Society of Cardiology (ESC) guidelines).

Finally, among thiazides, metolazone is usually reserved in the management of refractory heart failure patients as an adjunct to intravenous loop diuretics.

14.4 Loop diuretics

These rapidly acting agents are available in both oral and intravenous preparations. They are mostly used in the treatment of heart failure and are more efficacious in subjects with impaired renal profile, compared to thiazides. Generally, loop diuretics have a much wider dosage range (Table 14.1), and the effective dose in each individual patient is determined to a large extent by underlying renal function, with higher doses required for a similar response as the GFR declines. Torsemide and bumetanide have excellent oral bioavailability, whilst the bioavailability of oral furosemide is about 50% that of the intravenous route. With normal renal function, 40 mg of furosemide is equipotent to 1 mg of bumetanide and 20 mg of torsemide.

14.4.1 Mechanism of action

Loop diuretics block the Na^+/potassium (K^+)/Cl^- transport system in the thick part of the ascending loop of Henle (Figure 14.1). This results in increased luminal concentration of sodium, potassium, magnesium, and calcium, and consequently fluid diuresis. In addition to this, they also enhance prostaglandin-mediated venodilation, resulting in fluid redistribution and reduced cardiac preload, thus improving the symptoms of cardiac failure. An important concept in using loop diuretics is that of the so-called threshold dose. Little or no diuretic effect is seen below the threshold dose, which, in turn, depends largely on renal function. For example, the threshold dose of furosemide might be 10 mg when given intravenously in a patient with normal renal function, but may be as high as 80 mg in someone with a GFR of <45 mL/min. Although there is a dose–response effect, with a moderate increase in diuresis with doses above the threshold dose, there is also a ceiling dose, above which there is little further increase in fractional sodium excretion.

14.4.2 Contraindications, adverse effects, and drug interactions

- As with thiazides, most common side effects relate to excessive diuresis and metabolic disturbance. Hypokalaemia, hypocalcaemia, hypomagnesaemia, hypochloraemia, and hypovolaemia can all occur.
- Loop diuretics should be avoided in pregnancy (teratogenicity), hepatic failure, hypokalaemia, hypotension, and drug hypersensitivity.
- Hyperosmolar non-ketotic coma can be precipitated in diabetics, and agranulocytosis may rarely occur.
- Furosemide reduces the threshold for nephrotoxicity caused by aminoglycosides and cephalosporins when used concomitantly. It may also increase serum lithium levels and rapidly precipitate toxicity.

Table 14.1 Pharmacokinetics of thiazides and other diuretics

Diuretic	Dosing	Pharmacokinetics		Important considerations
		Oral bioavailability (%)	Elimination half-life (hours)	
Thiazide and thiazide-like diuretics				
Bendroflumethiazide	2.5–5 mg OD	100	5–9	Prefer CTD/IND over HCTZ
Hydrochlorothiazide	12.5–50 mg OD	65–75	6–15	Monitor electrolytes when initiating, changing dose, or symptomatic
Chlorthalidone	12.5–50 mg OD	60–70	40–60	
Indapamide	1.25–5 mg OD	>90	48–72	
Metolazone	2.5–20 mg daily	Approximately 65	14	
Loop diuretics				
Furosemide	20–600 mg daily (>80 mg doses, divide 2–3 times/day)	Approximately 60–65	1–2	Used for hypertension exclusively in advanced CKD with oedema
Torsemide	5–200 mg daily (>50 mg doses, divide twice daily)	>80	3–4	Demonstrate 'threshold effect'
Bumetanide	0.5–30 mg (>4 mg doses, divide 2–3 times/day)	>80	1–1.5	
Potassium-sparing and aldosterone antagonists				
Triamterene	50–300 mg divided BID	50–55	1.5–2.5	Used largely as adjunct with thiazide/loop diuretics to prevent hypokalaemia
Amiloride	5–10 mg BID	50	6–9	
Spironolactone	12.5–50 mg OD (may use 100 mg in hyperaldosteronism)	90	12–24	Used primarily in primary hyperaldosteronism or resistant HTN
Eplerenone	50–100 mg OD/BID	70	3–6	Monitor serum potassium 2 weeks after initiating therapy, especially in patients with CKD or those taking ACEI/ARB

OD, once daily; CTD, chlorthalidone; IND, indapamide; HCTZ, hydrochlorthiazide; CKD, chronic kidney disease; BID, twice daily; HTN, hypertension; ACEI, angiotensin-converting enzyme inhibitor; ARB, angiotensin receptor blocker.

14.4.3 Indications

Loop diuretics are most often indicated in the treatment of decompensated heart failure, often intravenously initially. Though used in the past for emergency treatment of blood pressure in hypertensive crises, most authorities now recommend alternatives. In the context of hypertension, the role of loop diuretics is largely restricted to those with advanced renal disease (GFR <45 mL/min) and concomitant oedema (from renal disease or heart failure). In these patients, initial therapy with loop diuretics may be preferred, followed by other agents (ACEIs or CCBs) once oedema is controlled.

14.5 Potassium-sparing diuretics and mineralocorticoid (aldosterone) antagonists

Spironolactone (an aldosterone receptor antagonist), eplerenone (a selective mineralocorticoid receptor antagonist), and amiloride (an epithelial sodium channel (ENaC) blocker) are all weak diuretics, better known for their potassium-sparing effects. They have an important role as adjuncts in the treatment of heart failure and refractory hypertension, and also in portal hypertension secondary to liver cirrhosis.

14.5.1 Mechanism of action

In response to reduced renal perfusion ensuing from decreased cardiac output, hypotension, or ischaemia, the juxtaglomerular cells increase secretion of renin (Figure 14.2). In addition, enhanced sodium diuresis and beta adrenergic stimulation can both increase renin secretion. Renin converts angiotensinogen to angiotensin I. This, in turn, is converted to the potent vasoconstrictor angiotensin II by ACE in the lungs. Angiotensin II stimulates aldosterone secretion by the adrenal glands. Aldosterone is a vasoconstrictor, enhances sodium reabsorption, and promotes potassium excretion.

Spironolactone inhibits aldosterone receptors located in the collecting tubule, resulting in decreased reabsorption of sodium and reduced excretion of potassium, helping with diuresis whilst retaining potassium. Eplerenone is a newer aldosterone antagonist derived from spironolactone and much more selective for the mineralocorticoid receptor, and does not possess the anti-androgen, anti-glucocorticoid, or anti-oestrogenic effects seen with spironolactone. The other potassium-sparing agents amiloride and triamterene interact with lumen membrane transporters to prevent urinary sodium entry into the cytoplasm. They are both direct inhibitors of potassium secretion.

14.5.2 Contraindications, adverse effects, and interactions

- Metabolic disturbances such as hyperkalaemia and hyponatraemia are not uncommon. Regular monitoring is advisable.

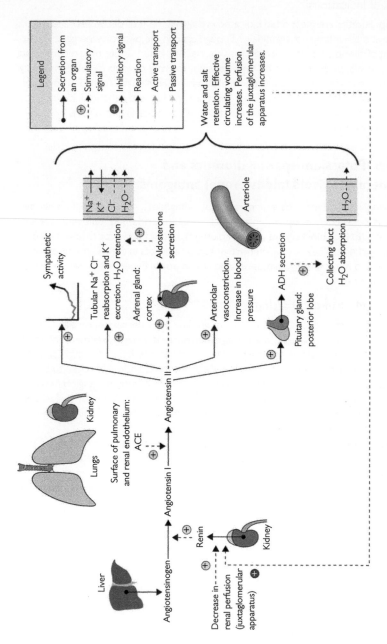

Figure 14.2 The renin–angiotensin–aldosterone cascade.

NaHCO₃, sodium bicarbonate; NA, sodium ions; K⁺, potassium ions; H₂O, water; ADH, antidiuretic hormone; Cl⁻, chloride; ACE, angiotensin converting enzyme.

- Gynaecomastia in men (which may be painful) and menstrual irregularities in perimenopausal women are relatively common side effects with spironolactone.
- Triamterene is contraindicated in patients with a history of renal calculi. In addition, concomitant use of non-steroidal anti-inflammatory drugs (NSAIDs) and triamterene is best avoided as this precipitates renal failure.
- Diuretics of any class are best avoided if the GFR is <20 mL/min.
- Aspirin may antagonize the effects of spironolactone.

14.5.3 Indications and uses

The potassium-sparing diuretics acting via ENaC blockade (i.e., triamterene and amiloride) have never been tested as sole agents for treatment of hypertension. Hence, these are almost solely reserved for combined use with loop/thiazide diuretics to prevent hypokalaemia, either in patients who demonstrate recurrent hypokalaemia with loops/thiazide diuretics or in cases where hypokalaemia must be avoided at all costs. In this regard, aldosterone antagonists (discussed below) may be a better choice because of now well-demonstrated additive blood pressure-lowering efficacy, as well as improvement in clinical outcomes in selected patient populations. If used due to intolerable side effects with aldosterone antagonists, amiloride is better tolerated than triamterene, which is a potential nephrotoxin, causing crystalluria and urinary cast formation in up to half of patients.

Aldosterone antagonists are not recommended as sole agents for hypertension of any severity. However, they have now well-proven efficacy:

- In patients with primary aldosteronism (drugs of choice)
- In patients with resistant hypertension (i.e. those with blood pressure not at goal despite optimal doses of three antihypertensives of different classes which should include a diuretic, an ACEI or angiotensin receptor blocker (ARB), and a CCB as evidenced by the Prevention and Treatment of hypertension with algorithm based therapy-2 trial (PATHWAY-2 trial, Anglo-Scandinavian Cardiac Outcomes Trial (ASCOT) observational study, Addition of spironolactone in patients with resistant arterial hypertension (ASPIRANT trial)
- In lieu of triamterene/amiloride as a potassium-sparing agent combined with a thiazide, or to potentiate the effects of loop diuretics in treatment of heart failure.

Eplerenone can be used instead of spironolactone in patients with intolerable adverse effects with the latter (e.g. gynaecomastia). However, it is less potent than spironolactone and requires twice-daily dosing to be effective. Besides the above indications in hypertension, aldosterone antagonists have now proven themselves effective in reducing symptom burden, as well as improving clinical outcomes, in patients who have heart failure with reduced ejection fraction (randomized aldactone evaluation study [RALES], Eplerenone Post–Acute Myocardial Infarction Heart Failure Efficacy and Survival Study [EPHESUS], and The Eplerenone in Mild patients hospitalisation and survival study in heart failure [EMPHASIS-HF] trials). They are now strongly recommended (class I recommendation) in patients who remain symptomatic (New York Heart Association class II–IV symptoms) despite standard-of-care treatment with beta blockers and ACEIs.

14.6 Conclusion

Diuretics continue to play an important and multifaceted role in the treatment of hypertension. Easy availability, cost-effectiveness, and a favourable safety profile ensure high compliance, whether used alone or as combination therapy. Importantly, diuretics may have a significant role in management of other coexisting conditions such as congestive cardiac failure and some causes of secondary hypertension (e.g. hyperaldosteronism). However, their use as first-line agents in the past has, to some extent, been subjugated by ACEIs and CCBs. Nevertheless, they remain well-proven agents to reduce cardiovascular events, heart failure, and mortality, and a viable option to be considered in combination with either CCBs or ACEIs, especially when significant hypervolaemia exists, for example, in heart failure, moderate renal disease, cirrhosis, etc.

KEY REFERENCES

Bazoukis G, Thomopoulos C, Tsioufis C (2018). Effect of mineralocorticoid antagonists on blood pressure lowering: overview and meta-analysis of randomized controlled trials in hypertension. *J Hypertens* **36**:987–94.

Beckett NS, Peters R, Fletcher AE, *et al.* (2008). Treatment of hypertension in patients 80 years of age or older. *N Engl J Med* **358**:1887–98.

Engberink RHGO, Frenkel WJ, Van Den Bogaard B, *et al.* (2015). Effects of thiazide-type and thiazide-like diuretics on cardiovascular events and mortality: systematic review and meta-analysis. *Hypertension* **65**:1033–40.

Jamerson KA, Weber MA, Bakris GL, *et al.* (2008). Benazepril plus amlodipine or hydrochlorothiazide for hypertension in high-risk patients. *N Engl J Med* **359**:2417–28.

Kostis JB, Wilson AC, Freudenberger RS, Cosgrove NM, Pressel SL, Davis BR (2005). Long-term effect of diuretic-based therapy on fatal outcomes in subjects with isolated systolic hypertension with and without diabetes. *Am J Cardiol* **95**:29–35.

National Institute for Health and Care Excellence (2018). Chronic heart failure in adults: diagnosis and management. NICE guideline [NG106]. Available from: https://www.nice.org.uk/guidance/ng106

National Institute for Health and Care Excellence (2019). Hypertension in adults: diagnosis and management. NICE guideline [NG136]. Available from: https://www.nice.org.uk/guidance/ng136

Václavík J, Sedlák R, Plachý M, et al. (2011). Addition of spironolactone in patients with resistant arterial hypertension (ASPIRANT): a randomized, double-blind, placebo-controlled trial. *Hypertension* **57**:1069–75.

Whelton PK, Carey RM, Aronow WS, et al. (2018). 2017 CC/AHA/AAPA/ABC/ACPM/AGS/APhA/ASH/ASPC/NMA/PCNA Guideline for the prevention, detection, evaluation, and management of high blood pressure in adults: a report of the American College of Cardiology/American Heart Association Task Force on Clinical Practice Guidelines. *J Am Coll Cardiol* **71**:e127–248.

Williams B, Macdonald TM, Morant S, et al. (2015). Spironolactone versus placebo, bisoprolol, and doxazosin to determine the optimal treatment for drug-resistant hypertension (PATHWAY-2): a randomised, double-blind, crossover trial. *Lancet* **386**:2059–68.

Williams B, Mancia G, Spiering W, et al. (2018). 2018 ESC/ESH Guidelines for the management of arterial hypertension. *Eur Heart J* **39**:3021–104.

Yancy CW, Jessup M, Bozkurt B, et al. (2017). 2017 ACC/AHA/HFSA Focused Update of the 2013 ACCF/AHA Guideline for the management of heart failure: a report of the American College of Cardiology/American Heart Association Task Force on Clinical Practice Guidelines and the Heart Failure Society of America. *J Am Coll Cardiol* **70**:776–803.

CHAPTER 15

Beta blockers in hypertension

Hatim Al-Lawati

KEY POINTS

- Beta blockers act by blocking beta adrenergic receptors in the body.
- Previously, they were an acceptable first-line, monotherapeutic agents for the treatment of hypertension.
- Contemporary clinical evidence suggests that they are not as effective as other classes of antihypertensive drugs in lowering blood pressure and reducing the overall cardiovascular and cerebrovascular risk.
- Current practice guidelines suggest that beta blockers should be reserved for use in the presence of other compelling indications such as ischaemic heart disease, heart failure, or concurrent arrhythmias.

15.1 Types of beta blockers

Beta blockers are classified based on their pharmacological properties—namely, their receptor selectivity, intrinsic sympathomimetic activity, associated alpha receptor blockade, and additional unique properties such as peripheral vasodilatation (nebivolol). Table 15.1 lists common beta blockers based on these properties.

15.2 Mechanism of action

Beta blockers inhibit the action of endogenous catecholamines (adrenaline and noradrenaline) on beta-1, beta-2, and beta-3 adrenergic receptors. Beta-1 adrenergic receptors are concentrated mainly in the heart and kidneys. Beta-2 receptors are located mainly in the lungs, gastrointestinal tract, liver, vascular smooth muscle, and skeletal muscle, whereas beta-3 adrenergic receptors are found in adipose tissue.

In the heart, beta-1 receptor blockade causes a negative chronotropic and inotropic effect, leading to decreased cardiac conduction velocity and intrinsic automaticity, as well as decreased cardiac contractility. Stimulation of beta-1 receptors in the kidney triggers renin release. A primary association between the antihypertensive effect of beta blockers and plasma renin activity is not well established. However, a significant reduction in blood pressure is noted with beta blockers in patients with high pre-treatment renin levels. Stimulation of beta-2 receptors induces smooth muscle relaxation, resulting in vasodilatation

Table 15.1 Various beta blockers and their properties

Drug	Beta-1 selectivity	Intrinsic sympathomimetic activity	Lipid solubility	Alpha blockade
Acebutolol	+	+	+	−
Atenolol	++	−	−	−
Betaxolol	++	−	−	−
Bisoprolol	+++	−	+	−
Bucindolol	−	−	+	−
Carteolol	−	+	−	−
Carvedilol	−	−	+++	+
Celiprolol	++	+	−	−
Esmolol	++	−	−	−
Labetalol	−	−	++	+
Metoprolol	++	−	++	−
Nadolol	−	−	+	−
Nebivolol	++	−	++	−
Penbutolol	−	+	+++	−
Pindolol	−	+++	++	−
Propranolol	−	−	+++	−
Sotalol	−	−	+	−
Timolol	−	−	++	−

and bronchodilation. They were once considered contraindicated in hypertension, due to concerns regarding vasoconstriction and consequently worsening of hypertension from beta-2 receptor blockade. However, subsequent studies disproved this theory. Patients receiving propranolol in doses varying from 30 to 400 mg per day had, on average, a 19 mmHg fall in the systolic value and a 7 mmHg reduction in the diastolic value of the supine blood pressure reading.

The antihypertensive effect of beta blockers therefore can be summarized in the following mechanisms:

- Reduction in cardiac output (due to negative chronotropic and inotropic effects)
- Reduction in renin release from the kidneys, and
- Reduction in the central nervous system sympathetic activity.

15.3 Clinical evidence on the role of beta blockers in hypertension

Early placebo-controlled studies proved that beta blockers are effective in reducing blood pressure. However, this was not associated with a reduction in morbidity or mortality. Their use in hypertension therefore needs to be carefully appraised in patients with or without other compelling indications such as ischaemic heart disease, heart failure, chronic kidney disease, and cerebrovascular disease, in elderly patients and in ethnic minorities, etc.

Despite the dearth of clinical evidence confirming the beneficial effects of beta blockers, these drugs and diuretics were considered first-line antihypertensive therapy in the period from 1983 to 1997. More recent guidelines (see Chapter 11) do not endorse this approach due to lack of effectiveness in lowering blood pressure and in preventing adverse clinical outcomes.

Clinical trials have repeatedly shown that beta blockers are inferior to other agents in reducing blood pressure. Blood pressure control was achieved in <50% of patients randomized to atenolol in the Losartan Intervention For Endpoint reduction in hypertension (LIFE) trial and <10% of the patients remained on beta blocker monotherapy. In the first Swedish Trial in Old Patients with Hypertension (STOP-Hypertension 1), blood pressure control was half as effective with beta blockers, as compared to diuretics. In the Anglo-Scandinavian Cardiac Outcomes Trial-Blood Pressure Lowering Arm (ASCOT-BPLA) study, patients treated with an amlodipine-based regimen had a mean additional 1.7 mmHg reduction in systolic blood pressure and a 2.0 mmHg reduction in diastolic blood pressure, as compared to an atenolol-based treatment. The seemingly trivial numerical between-group difference was associated with a significant 23% relative reduction in the risk of stroke and a 14% relative reduction in coronary events, favouring the amlodipine-treated group.

In the Medical Research Council (MRC) study, diuretic therapy was associated with a lower risk of cardiovascular events, compared to beta blockers, independent of the magnitude of decrease in blood pressure. This observation has major implications. It is either that diuretics confer additional benefits independent of the decrease in arterial pressure or the possibility that beta blockers confer an ill-effect on the cardiovascular well-being of elderly patients that overrides the potential benefits derived from the antihypertensive effect.

Beta blockers are less effective in controlling the central aortic pressure, as compared to peripheral brachial pressure measurements. In the Conduit Artery Functional Endpoint (CAFE) study, for the same peripheral arterial blood pressure, atenolol/bendroflumethiazide-based treatment resulted in a 4.3 mmHg higher central aortic systolic blood pressure and a 3 mmHg higher central aortic pulse pressure, compared to amlodipine/perindopril-based treatment.

A 2012 Cochrane review by Wiysonge and colleagues demonstrated that beta blockers are inferior to calcium channel blockers in reducing all-cause mortality, stroke, and total cardiovascular events, and to renin–angiotensin system inhibition in decreasing stroke. Similar findings were reported by Lindholm and colleagues. In another meta-analysis, Khan and McAlister (2006) found beta blockers to be inferior to all other therapies in decreasing a composite outcome of major cardiovascular events (stroke, myocardial infarction, and death) and stroke in elderly hypertensive patients. The same was observed in younger patients. All investigators concluded that current available evidence does not support the use of beta blockers as first-line drugs in the treatment of hypertension.

Perhaps the largest meta-analysis to date was by Thomopoulos and colleagues (2020) which included data from 84 randomized controlled trials, accumulating 542,330 patient-years' follow-up. It compared beta blockers to placebo and other antihypertensive agents. When compared to placebo, beta blockers resulted in a 22% relative reduction in risk of combined endpoint of stroke, coronary heart disease, and heart failure, with no effect on mortality. However, they were substantially less protective against stroke and all-cause mortality, when compared to other agents, with a reported relative increase of 6% in mortality and 21% in stroke. This was consistent with previously published systematic reviews and meta-analyses reporting an alarming 24–30% increase in stroke events with beta blockers, compared to calcium channel blockers and inhibitors of the renin–angiotensin–aldosterone system (RAAS), with the risk being greatest in elderly patients (Tables 15.2 and 15.3).

Based on available evidence, recent guidelines issued by the European Society of Hypertension and the European Society of Cardiology do not discourage the use of beta blockers. These agents can still be first-line antihypertensive agents, owing to reported benefits in patients post-myocardial infarction or those with heart failure or young women planning pregnancy. However, they do caution

Table 15.2 Overview of major meta-analyses of randomized controlled trials of beta blockers in patients with hypertension versus placebo

Meta-analysis	Number of trials	Mortality	Myocardial infarction	Stroke
Thomopoulos et al., 2020	67	0.95 (0.84–1.06)	0.88 (0.77–1.01)	0.77 (0.61–0.97)
Wiysonge et al., 2007	4	0.99 (0.88–1.11)	0.93 (0.81–1.07)	0.80 (0.66–0.96)
Bradley et al., 2006	4	0.99 (0.88–1.11)	0.93 (0.81–1.07)	0.80 (0.66–0.96)
Khan et al., 2006	5	0.91 (0.74–1.12)	0.98 (0.83–1.16)	0.78 (0.63–0.98)
Lindholm et al., 2005	7	0.95 (0.86–1.04)	0.93 (0.83–1.05)	0.81 (0.71–0.93)
Carlberg et al., 2004 (atenolol)	4	1.01 (0.89–1.15)	0.99 (0.83–1.19)	0.85 (0.72–1.01)

Numbers represent the hazard ratio (HR) (95% confidence interval).

Table 15.3 Overview of major meta-analyses of randomized controlled trials of beta blockers in patients with hypertension versus other antihypertensive agents

Meta-analysis	No. of trials	Mortality	Myocardial infarction	Stroke
Thomopoulos et al., 2020	24	1.06 (1.01–1.12)	1.01 (0.93–1.12)	1.21 (1.07–1.38)
Khan et al., 2006	5	0.97 (0.83–1.14)	0.97 (0.86–1.10)	0.99 (0.67–1.44)
Khan et al., 2006	7	1.05 (0.99–1.11)	1.06 (0.94–1.20)	1.18 (1.07–1.30)
Lindholm et al., 2005	13	1.03 (0.99–1.08)	1.02 (0.93–1.12)	1.16 (1.04–1.30)
Carlberg et al., 2004 (atenolol)	5	1.13 (0.97–1.33)	1.0 (0.89–1.20)	1.30 (1.12–1.50)

Numbers represent the hazard ratio (HR) (95% confidence interval).

healthcare providers regarding possible weight gain and other unfavourable metabolic effects. This class is best avoided in patients with multiple cardiovascular risk factors, including the metabolic syndrome and associated conditions that make the risk of incident diabetes higher—namely, abdominal obesity, impaired fasting glucose, and impaired glucose tolerance.

15.4 Beta blockers and ischaemic heart disease

Ischaemic heart disease is the most common form of target organ damage associated with hypertension. Beta blockers are an automatic first choice in hypertensive patients with stable angina pectoris. Alternatively, calcium channel blockers may be used to circumvent some of the adverse effects of beta blockers on insulin sensitivity, weight control, exercise tolerance, and sexual function.

Beta blockers reduce mortality in patients with prior myocardial infarction. Analyses from prospective randomized trials reported a 23% mortality reduction, compared to up to 40% in observational studies. The number needed to treat over 1 year is 84 patients to prevent one death, and 107 patients to prevent one non-fatal reinfarction. Evidently, the impact on mortality reduction is far lower with beta blockers than with antiplatelet agents or statins.

In patients with acute myocardial infarction (AMI), early treatment with intravenous beta blockers produced mixed outcomes. In the Thrombolysis In Myocardial Infarction trial, phase II-B (TIMI-2B), intravenous metoprolol given within 2 hours of thrombolytic therapy resulted in lower mortality at 6 days and fewer reinfarction and recurrent anginal events. However, it did not influence left ventricular ejection fraction (LVEF) at discharge, the primary study endpoint. The First International Study of Infarct Survival (ISIS-1) demonstrated a significant reduction in mortality mostly in the first 24 hours, but also at 1 week and 1 year, when patients with suspected AMI were treated with atenolol within 24 hours of symptom onset. The Metoprolol In Acute Myocardial Infarction (MIAMI) study showed a 30% mortality reduction with early initiation of intravenous metoprolol in high-risk patients and significantly fewer episodes of ventricular and supraventricular arrhythmias. In contrast, a prospective post hoc analysis from the Global Utilization of Streptokinase and Tissue Plasminogen Activator for Occluded Coronary Arteries (GUSTO-1) trial showed that early intravenous atenolol resulted in 30% increased risk in 30-day deaths, along with a greater incidence of heart failure, shock, and pacemaker use. The more recent, and largest to date, Clopidogrel and Metoprolol in Myocardial Infarction Trial/Second Chinese Cardiac Study (COMMIT-CCS-2) showed that even though early intravenous metoprolol was associated with a significant reduction in reinfarction rates and ventricular fibrillation, the benefit was offset by a significant 30% increase in the risk of cardiogenic shock in the first 24 hours, especially in haemodynamically tenuous patients.

15.5 Heart failure and beta blockers

Beta blockers were initially considered detrimental in heart failure owing to their negative inotropic effect. However, large-scale randomized controlled trials, such as the Cardiac Insufficiency Bisoprolol Study II (CIBIS-II), the Metoprolol CR/XL Randomised Intervention Trial in Congestive Heart Failure (MERIT-HF) study, and the US Carvedilol Heart Failure Study, were terminated early, given significant reduction in overall mortality, sudden death, and death due to worsening heart failure with use of beta blockers in symptomatic chronic heart failure secondary to left ventricular systolic dysfunction. Multiple meta-analyses have clearly shown that mortality benefit occurred irrespective of gender, age, and presence or absence of diabetes.

In heart failure with preserved ejection fraction, beta blockers, by virtue of their negative chronotropic effects, prolong diastole, potentially improving the haemodynamic response to exercise. Anecdotal evidence indicates that propranolol can reduce mortality and left ventricular mass in patients with heart failure symptoms and prior myocardial infarction, but with preserved left ventricular systolic function. However, there is no significant improvement in radionuclide parameters of left ventricular diastolic relaxation, as shown in a study of patients with moderate systolic heart failure treated with carvedilol versus placebo. Using echocardiographic parameters, Pallazouli and colleagues (2004) showed that carvedilol therapy altered diastolic filling favourably—the restrictive transmitral Doppler filling pattern regressed to a 'pseudonormal' pattern after 6 months of carvedilol. Larger-scale investigations would be necessary to confirm these findings.

15.6 Beta blockers and diabetes

Beta blockers increase insulin resistance predisposing to diabetes. In a meta-analysis of 22 clinical trials, the risk of diabetes with beta blockers and diuretics was much higher than with placebo. In another large meta-analysis of 12 studies evaluating 94,492 patients, beta blocker therapy resulted in a 22% relative increase in the risk of incident diabetes, compared to non-diuretic antihypertensive agents. A higher baseline body mass index and fasting blood glucose levels were significant predictors of new-onset diabetes mellitus. The risk was greater with atenolol and in the elderly.

Possible mechanisms leading to development of diabetes include weight gain, attenuation of beta receptor-mediated release of insulin from pancreatic beta cells, and decreased blood flow in skeletal muscle tissue leading to decreased insulin sensitivity. Beta blockers can also produce hypoglycaemia unawareness because of their suppressive effect on the autonomic system.

In the Glycemic Effect of Diabetes Mellitus: Carvedilol-Metoprolol Comparison In Hypertensives (GEMINI) trial, there was an increase in the on-treatment HbA1c with metoprolol, but not with carvedilol, suggesting that it is not a class effect.

15.7 Effect of beta blockers on left ventricular hypertrophy

Left ventricular hypertrophy (LVH) remains a powerful predictor of cardiovascular mortality and morbidity. Its regression reduces that risk, irrespective of the degree of blood pressure reduction. A meta-analysis on the effects of various antihypertensive therapies on LVH regression found beta blockers to be inferior to diuretics, calcium channel antagonists, angiotensin-converting enzyme (ACE) inhibitors, and angiotensin receptor blockers (ARBs). In the LIFE study, treatment with losartan resulted in greater LVH regression, as compared to atenolol for the same degree of blood pressure reduction.

15.8 Beta blockers and weight gain

Beta blocker therapy causes a small, but consistent, weight gain. This observation was reported in only a minority of clinical trials which monitored weight changes during treatment. In these, beta blockers were associated with a 1.2 kg weight gain (0.4–3.5 kg). This was attributed to a reduction in the metabolic rate and also to their negative effect on energy metabolism. Obesity management in overweight, hypertensive patients may therefore be more challenging with beta blocker treatment.

15.9 Beta blockers in black patients

The prevalence, severity, and impact of hypertension is greater in black patients, who also demonstrate an attenuated overall blood pressure response to monotherapy with beta blockers, ACE inhibitors, or ARBs, compared to diuretics or calcium channel blockers. In black patients, beta blockers were equivalent to placebo in their blood pressure-lowering effect. Furthermore, there are reports of aggravated systolic hypertension in this unique group of patients. Therefore, once proven ineffective, beta blocker therapy should be discontinued, rather than continue with further dose escalation.

15.10 Beta blockers in pregnant women

Beta blockers have been used in pregnancy to treat hypertension and thyrotoxicosis and for rate control in atrial fibrillation. Their pharmacodynamic properties have been well elucidated in the pregnant state. Serious maternal side effects are rare. Fetal pharmacodynamics and fetal side effects are less well known. The literature is, at times, contradictory. The safety profile of these agents, particularly atenolol and propranolol, is somewhat controversial because of individual reports of adverse effects on the fetus.

A meta-analysis of 13 trials including 1480 women compared beta blockers with placebo and showed that beta blocker therapy reduced the risk of severe hypertension and the need for additional antihypertensives. The analysis was too constrained to generate conclusions pertaining to perinatal mortality or preterm birth. Beta blockers also seem to be associated with an increase in small-for-gestational-age (SGA) infants. They were compared to methyldopa in 11 trials and appeared to be more effective and probably equally safe. Labetalol, a beta blocker with alpha-blocking properties, is commonly used in pregnancy.

15.11 Beta blockers and their effect on quality of life

Beta blockers have been reported to adversely impact normal exercise capacity, cognitive function, sleep quality, overall mood, and sexual function (erectile failure in men and depressed libido in both sexes). Furthermore, studies have reported memory impairment, particularly with non-selective lipophilic beta blockers (such as propranolol), which, in addition to cognitive impairment, inhibit rapid eye movement sleep and negatively influence sleep quality.

Large-scale population studies have demonstrated an increase in the use of antidepressant medications within 12 months of prescribing a beta blocker, as compared to a reference group of patients treated for chronic diseases. However, such associations were frequently confounded and in one double-blind, randomized controlled crossover study, there appeared to be no significant effect on cognitive function.

Beta blocker therapy is implicated in sexual dysfunction, both by a depressant effect on male erection and more generally by decreased libido. There have been several crossover studies reporting a significant reduction in sexual activity in hypertensive men on beta blockers, compared to active controls such as lisinopril or valsartan. Unfortunately, these do not address the mechanical or psychosexual nature of the dysfunction. Several hypotheses have been proposed to rationalize this effect, including reduction in the levels of testosterone in males. However, the studies are far from definitive and have always failed to correlate with objective sexual/erectile function assessment.

15.12 Third-generation beta blockers

Third-generation beta blockers are characterized by their vasodilatory activity and are more promising in their clinical effects. Nebivolol is a third-generation lipophilic beta blocker with distinct beta-1 selective and vasodilatory properties. In ex vivo and human studies, nebivolol increased the bioavailability of nitric oxide (NO), resulting in vasodilatation and enhanced endothelial function. In addition, it carries antioxidant properties. It results in a greater reduction in central aortic pressure in humans, compared to atenolol. The pharmacological profile is unique due to the significant antihypertensive effect from lowering of both cardiac pre-load and afterload, making it also potentially beneficial in patients with heart failure. The randomized trial to determine the effect of nebivolol on mortality and cardiovascular hospital admission in elderly patients with heart failure (SENIORS) demonstrated a significant reduction in all-cause mortality and cardiovascular hospital admissions in elderly patients with heart failure. In general, nebivolol is well tolerated and lacks significant influence on glucose or plasma lipid metabolism. It is also devoid of any intrinsic sympathomimetic activity (ISA).

15.13 Contraindications

Some of the absolute contraindications to beta blockers include severe asthma and obstructive airways disease. These agents may induce or exacerbate bronchospasm, heart blocks and bradyarrhythmias, and hypotension and shock.

They should be used with caution in patients with severely decompensated heart failure, peripheral vascular disease, and poorly controlled insulin-dependent diabetes. Selective agents are best avoided in patients suspected to have phaeochromocytoma, as unopposed alpha adrenergic agonist action may lead to a serious hypertensive crisis.

KEY REFERENCES

Bangalore S, Messerli FH, Kostis JB, et al. (2007). Cardiovascular protection using beta-blockers: a critical review of the evidence. J Am Coll Cardiol 50:563–72.

Bradley HA, Wiysonge CS, Volmink JA, et al. (2006). How strong is the evidence for use of beta-blockers as first-line therapy for hypertension? Systematic review and meta-analysis. J Hypertens 24:2131–41.

Brewster LM, van Montfrans GA, Kleijnen J (2004). Systematic review: antihypertensive drug therapy in black patients. Ann Intern Med 141:614–27.

Carlberg B, Samuelsson O, Lindholm LH (2004). Atenolol in hypertension: is it a wise choice? Lancet 364:1684–9.

COMMIT Collaborative Group (2005). Early intravenous then oral metopolol in 45,852 patients with acute myocardial infarction: a randomized placebo-controlled trial. *Lancet* **366**:1622–32.

Khan N, McAlister FA. (2006). Re-examining the efficacy of beta-blockers for the treatment of hypertension: a meta-analysis. *CMAJ* **174**(12):1737–42. doi:10.1503/cmaj.060110. Erratum in: *CMAJ* 176(7):976.

Larochelle P, Tobe SV, Lacourciere Y (2014). Beta blockers in hypertension: studies and meta-analyses over the years. *Can J Cardiol* **30**(5 suppl):S16–22.

Lindholm LH, Carlberg B, Samuelsson O (2005). Should beta blockers remain first choice in treatment of primary hypertension? A meta-analysis. *Lancet* **366**:1545–53.

Messerli FH, Grossman E, Goldbourt U (1998). Are beta-blockers efficacious as first-line therapy for hypertension in the elderly? A systematic review. *JAMA* **279**:1903–7.

Thomopoulos C, Bazoukis G, Tsioufis C, Mancia G (2020). Beta-blockers in hypertension: overview and meta-analysis of randomized outcome trials. *J Hypertens* **38**:1669–81.

Wiysonge CS, Bradley H, Volmink J, et al. (2012). Beta-blockers for hypertension. *Cochrane Database Syst Rev* **15**:CD002003.

CHAPTER 15

CHAPTER 16

Calcium channel blockers in hypertension

Stephanie Lip and Sandosh Padmanabhan

KEY POINTS

- Calcium channel blockers are a biochemically heterogenous group of drugs that are very effective in lowering blood pressure.
- Clinical trials have demonstrated their use results in improved cardiovascular outcomes in patients at high cardiovascular risk.
- Current guidelines recommend that these agents are used as first-line drugs in the treatment of hypertension.
- Calcium channel blockers are generally well tolerated.

16.1 Introduction

Calcium channel blockers (CCBs) are an effective antihypertensive drug class for hypertension management and features among the first-line agents in all hypertension guidelines. The term was first coined by Fleckenstein in 1969 to describe a compound which showed negative inotropic and coronary vasodilatory properties, resulting from drug discovery programmes directed towards developing treatment for angina pectoris. A range of compounds were identified showing these properties, including diphenylmethylpiperazines (lidoflazine, cinnarizine, flunarizine), phenylalkylamines (verapamil), and dihydropyridines (nifedipine, nimodipine, nisoldipine). Verapamil was the first CCB licensed for clinical use.

16.2 Mechanism of action

CCBs inhibit cellular calcium influx through voltage-dependent calcium channels which, in turn, causes vasodilatation and reduces myocardial contractility. Although all CCBs share the common property of inhibiting cellular calcium influx, they possess differing effects on vascular smooth muscle, cardiac myocytes, and cardiac conductive tissue. CCBs are classified into dihydropyridines and non-dihydropyridines. Dihydropyridines bind preferentially to L-type calcium channels which are found in vascular smooth muscle and are predominantly vasodilators with limited inotropic and chronotropic effects. Non-dihydropyridines (benzothiazepine (diltiazem) and phenylalkylamine (verapamil)) predominantly act on L-type calcium channels found in the sinoatrial and atrioventricular node and hence slow cardiac contractility and conduction, with a less potent vasodilatory effect. Over the last decade, fourth-generation CCBs (cilnidipine and lercanidipine) have been developed, with effects on N-type calcium channels and associated with fewer side effects. CCBs are well absorbed orally, undergo high hepatic first-pass metabolism by cytochrome P450 (CYP3A4), and are renally excreted. The key characteristics of CCBs are summarized in Table 16.1.

16.3 Calcium channel blockers in hypertension

CCBs are recommended as first-line agents in the treatment of hypertension, either as single or combination therapy (National Institute for Health and Care Excellence (NICE), American College of Cardiology (ACC)/American Heart Association (AHA), European Society of Hypertension (ESH) Hypertension Guidelines). These recommendations are based on unequivocal evidence from several randomized clinical trials which have demonstrated the effectiveness and potency of CCBs in the management of hypertension and cardiovascular outcomes. A majority of randomized controlled trials (RCTs) demonstrating the benefits of CCBs on outcomes have used dihydropyridines (especially amlodipine), and a minority have studied non-dihydropyridines (verapamil and diltiazem). There is no substantial difference in effectiveness between dihydropyridines and non-dihydropyridines, compared to other antihypertensive drug classes. CCBs are recommended as first-line agents for hypertension in those of African ancestry and older (>55 years) patients. They have a greater effect on stroke reduction than expected for the blood pressure reduction achieved, but may also be less effective at preventing heart failure with reduced ejection fraction (HFrEF). Table 16.2 is a summary of the main clinical trials involving CCBs in hypertension management and cardiovascular outcomes.

16.4 Calcium channel blockers in other cardiovascular conditions

CCBs are used as an adjunctive therapy for patients with chronic stable angina who are already established on optimal therapy. It is used also in prevention of coronary spasm following coronary artery bypass grafting. The negative chronotropic effects of diltiazem and verapamil make them useful for rate control in supraventricular arrhythmias. In patients with hypertrophic cardiomyopathy, verapamil has been found to improve coronary vasomotor response to physical stress.

There is no evidence that CCBs reduce cardiovascular mortality in patients with acute myocardial infarction. Non-dihydropyridine CCBs are contraindicated in HFrEF, but safe to use in patients with heart failure with preserved ejection fraction. Short-acting nifedipine is contraindicated in the presence of ischaemic

Table 16.1 Characteristics of calcium channel blockers

Class	Dihydropyridines	Non-dihydropyridines	
Molecular structure	$C_6H_9O_3$ Amlodipine	Verapamil	• HCl Diltiazem
First generation	Nifedipine Nicardipine	Verapamil	Diltiazem
Second generation	Nifedipine extended-release Nimodipine Felodipine Benidipine* Isradipine*		
Third generation	Amlodipine Lacidipine Lercanidipine Azelnidipine* Barnidipine*		
Fourth generation	Cilnidipine*		
Target calcium channels	L-type N-type (amlodipine and cilnidipine) T-type (amlodipine, israpidine, nifedipine)	L-type, N-type, P/Q-type, T-type	L-type

* Not licensed in the United Kingdom.

Table 16.2 Summary of trial evidence for calcium channel blockers in hypertension

Trial (year of publication)	Trial design	Agents used and findings
Calcium channel blockers and blood pressure lowering		
VA Cooperative (1993)	1292 hypertensive patients Randomized, double-blind, placebo-controlled	Evaluated the efficacy of six common antihypertensive drugs versus placebo on BP lowering Diltiazem showed the highest treatment success rate, with 59% of treated hypertensive patients achieving BP goal at the end of the titration phase Diltiazem ranked first for younger blacks (<60 years) and older blacks (≥60 years), among whom the success rate was 64%
Valsartan Antihypertensive Long-term Use Evaluation (VALUE) trial (2006)	15,245 hypertensives with multiple additional risk factors Double-blind, active-controlled, parallel group	Evaluated outcomes in hypertensive subjects treated with valsartan- or amlodipine-based regimens Similar BP lowering in amlodipine and valsartan groups No difference in primary composite cardiac endpoints, stroke, myocardial infarction, and all-cause death, but significantly more heart failure in the amlodipine group
Calcium channel blockers and cardiovascular outcomes in hypertension		
Syst-Eur (1997)	4695 hypertensive patients, aged ≥60 years with isolated systolic hypertension	Nitrendipine demonstrated a greater reduction in blood pressure, compared to placebo, with 31% greater reduction in fatal and non-fatal strokes combined
Swedish Trial in Old Patients with Hypertension-2 (STOP-2) (1999)	6614 hypertensive patients (70–84 years) Randomized, open-label, blinded endpoint	Felodipine or israpidine versus conventional hypertensive agents (beta blocker, diuretic, ACE inhibitor, or calcium channel blocker) No difference when calcium channel blockers compared to diuretics/beta blockers or with ACE inhibitors. Blood pressure reduction was noted in all groups Risk of myocardial infarction and heart failure was lower in the ACE inhibitor group versus the CCB group

Table 16.2 Continued		
Trial (year of publication)	Trial design	Agents used and findings
International Nifedipine GITS Study of Intervention as a Goal in Hypertension Treatment (INSIGHT) (2000)	6321 hypertensives (55–80 years) with one additional cardiovascular risk factor and hypertension (BP ≥150/95 mmHg or ≥160 mmHg systolic) Prospective, randomized, double-blind	Nifedipine equivalent to co-amilozide in reducing cardiovascular mortality or cerebrovascular complications
NORdic DILtiazem (NORDIC) study (2000)	10,881 patients (50–74 years) with diastolic BP >100 mmHg Prospective, randomized, open-label, blinded endpoint	No difference between diltiazem, beta blocker, and diuretics for the primary outcome—all-cause and cardiovascular mortality (stroke, myocardial infarction, and other cardiovascular death)
Antihypertensive and Lipid Lowering to Prevent Heart Attack Trial (ALLHAT) (2002)	33,357 hypertensives with one additional cardiovascular risk factor	Amlodipine and lisinopril were equivalent to chlorthalidone in controlling high BP or reducing cardiovascular events Amlodipine had a 38% higher incidence of heart failure, compared to chlorthalidone Mean BP reduction in the amlodipine-treated group was 11.5 ± 9.3 mmHg, with 40% of patients requiring an additional agent(s) Systolic BP reduction was greater with chlorthalidone, compared to lisinopril or amlodipine
Controlled ONset Verapamil INvestigation of Cardiovascular Endpoints (CONVINCE) study (2003)	16,602 hypertensives with one additional cardiovascular risk factor	Verapamil (controlled-onset, extended-release (COER)) equivalent to atenolol in BP reduction (13.6 ± 7.8 mmHg for verapamil, compared to 13.5 ± 7.1 mmHg in the beta blocker group) and no observed difference in primary cardiovascular outcome between treatment groups

(continued)

Table 16.2 Continued

Trial (year of publication)	Trial design	Agents used and findings
International Verapamil SR Trandolapril Study (INVEST) (2003)	22,576 hypertensives with established coronary disease	Patients were randomized to either sustained-release verapamil with trandolapril and hydrochlorothiazide as stepped regimens or to twice-daily atenolol plus daily hydrochlorothiazide and trandolapril as stepped regimens No significant difference between treatment arms for BP reduction and cardiovascular outcomes
Anglo Scandinavian Cardiac Outcomes Trial–Blood Pressure Lowering Arm (ASCOT–BPLA) study (2005)	19,342 hypertensives with no previous coronary disease	The study was stopped prematurely after 5.5 years due to a significant reduction in all cause-mortality in the amlodipine and perindopril arms The amlodipine arm showed statistically significant reductions in all-cause mortality (11%), cardiovascular mortality, (24%), all strokes (23%)

BP, blood pressure; ACE, angiotensin-converting enzyme.

heart disease because of reflex tachycardia and hypotension. Long-acting dihydropyridines (amlodipine and felodipine) are safe to use in coronary artery disease or heart failure.

Nimodipine, which is not used to treat hypertension, is effective in improving outcomes in patients with aneurysmal subarachnoid haemorrhage by reducing vasospasm of cerebral flow. It is administered orally or intravenously.

16.5 Calcium channel blockers in non-cardiovascular conditions

16.5.1 Proteinuric nephropathy

Calcium channel antagonist groups also have a divergent role in renoprotection. In hypertensive patients with proteinuria (>300 mg of protein per gram of creatinine), use of dihydropyridine CCBs have failed to slow progression of nephropathy. If used as antihypertensive agents, they must be used in conjunction with angiotensin-converting enzyme (ACE) inhibitors or angiotensin II receptor antagonists. In contrast, a systematic review of 28 clinical trials by Bakris and colleagues (2004) suggested that whilst dihydropyridine and non-dihydropyridine calcium channel blockers are similarly efficacious at reducing blood pressure, non-dihydropyridine calcium channel blockers demonstrate greater reductions in proteinuria in patients with nephropathy (with or without diabetes).

16.5.2 Migraine

Verapamil has potential use for preventative therapy of migraine. However, the side effects of bradycardia and heart block need to be monitored. Flunarizine, a non-specific calcium channel blocker, has been used for migraine attacks.

16.5.3 Hyperaldosteronism

Inhibition of L-type calcium channels has been shown to inhibit aldosterone production in some studies. Somatic mutations in the genes encoding the L-type calcium channel have been identified in some patients with aldosterone-producing adenomas and primary aldosteronism. Increased calcium influx associated with these gain-of-function mutations is a sufficient stimulus for aldosterone production and cell proliferation in the adrenal glomerulosa. This raises the possibility of CCBs as targeted therapy to reduce aldosterone production in patients who harbour these mutations.

16.5.4 Cancer

Observational studies showed CCBs are associated with an increased incidence of breast cancer. However, this is not evident in RCTs involving CCBs. Conversely, CCBs are used as adjuvants to chemotherapy regimens for pancreatic, gastric, and lung cancers, based on their effects on cell proliferation and calcium influx from *in vitro* studies.

16.5.5 Bipolar disorder

Bipolar disorder is a common mental disorder, for which treatment is lithium and sodium valproate. Single nucleotide polymorphisms in *CACNA1C*, which encodes the L-type calcium channel, have been associated with bipolar disorder, raising the possibility of CCBs as a therapeutic option for this disease.

16.6 Adverse effects, safety, and tolerability

Common side effects reported by patients in the first weeks of commencing CCBs include flushing, peripheral oedema, hypotension, tachycardia, rash, headache, and constipation. Peripheral oedema is the most common side effect, which is usually dose-dependent, due to increased calcium channel blocker-mediated vasodilatation. Clinically significant peripheral oedema is an indication to discontinue CCBs or alternatively consider newer-generation CCBs, such as lercanidipine, which has a lower incidence of this side effect. If clinically warranted, addition of an ACE inhibitor can significantly reduce the severity of oedema because ACE inhibitor/angiotensin receptor blocker (ARB)-mediated vasodilatation can reduce transcapillary pressure. Addition of diuretics in the setting of CCB-induced peripheral oedema is not ideal, as it leads to unnecessary polypharmacy and causes potential harm in elderly patients. CCBs can also exacerbate gastro-oesophageal reflux symptoms, which is commonly seen with amlodipine use.

Non-dihydropyridines (verapamil, diltiazem) have side effects which are dose-dependent—constipation, bradycardia, and worsening cardiac output (due to negative inotropic effects), which can occur in 25% of patients. Thus, these drugs are contraindicated in patients on beta blockers and those with HFrEF and cardiac bradyarrhythmias (second- or third-degree atrioventricular block, sick sinus syndrome). Long-term use can lead to gingival hyperplasia in some patients.

Certain CCBs, such as amlodipine, diltiazem, felodipine, nicardipine, nifedipine, and verapamil, are relatively potent CYP3A4 inhibitors at clinically relevant doses. Drug–drug interactions could result after co-prescription of CYP3A4-metabolized statins (lovastatin, simvastatin, and atorvastatin) and CCBs that inhibit CYP3A4, resulting in increased blood levels of statins. Fluvastatin, pravastatin, and rosuvastatin are not metabolized by CYP3A4 to any significant extent and do not interact with CCBs. Though atorvastatin is also metabolized by CYP3A4, it is less susceptible to interaction with CYP3A4 inhibitors than simvastatin due to its structure, and current Medicines and Healthcare products Regulatory Agency (MHRA) recommendations only advise a reduction of the simvastatin dose if co-prescribed with amlodipine.

The role of CCBs in hypertension has not been without controversy. An increase in the incidence of acute myocardial infarction was observed in trials of nifedipine (short-acting), but not long-acting agents. An initial meta-analysis, which highlighted that these drugs are potentially dangerous if used long term, examined 27,743 patients in nine clinical trials, suggesting an increased risk of myocardial infarction, heart failure, and major cardiovascular events. This was felt to be due to profound hypotension and sympathetic activation induced by large doses of nifedipine in these haemodynamically unstable patient groups. This was repudiated by the Blood Pressure Lowering Treatment Trialists Collaboration which did not find any increased risk with use of CCBs. Further supportive evidence for the safety and efficacy of CCBs has been reported in three more recent meta-analyses—a further two reports from the Blood Pressure Lowering Treatment Trialists Collaboration, both examining 27 trials (136,124 patients in one and 158,709 patients, including 33,395 with diabetes, in the other); and Staesson and colleagues (2002) looking at nine trials (65,605 patients). These meta-analyses supported the safety and efficacy of CCBs in the reduction and prevention of major cardiovascular events.

There are newer CCBs that have improved tolerability and efficacy, compared to currently available CCBs. Besides lercanidipine, lacidipine is a long-acting dihydropyridine CCB with similar characteristics in randomized controlled trials, comparable incidence of cardiovascular events, and also a lower incidence of vasodilatory oedema. Another newer agent is azelnidipine (only approved in Japan).

16.7 Calcium channel blocker overdose

In patients who have taken a CCB overdose, hypotension and bradycardia are common features and can be life-threatening. Patients usually present asymptomatically initially and progress to having severe hypotension and cardiovascular collapse. A prognostic indicator is hyperglycaemia as beta islet cells of pancreas are dependent on calcium influx to release insulin and this is impaired in cases of overdose. Treatment requires level 2 care with aggressive fluid resuscitation, inotropic support, insulin for hyperglycaemia, cautious administration of intravenous calcium, and consideration of atropine in severe bradycardia.

16.8 Conclusion

CCBs are effective antihypertensive agents, and multiple clinical trial evidence points to their efficacy in treating hypertension, either as single agents or in conjunction with other antihypertensives. The recent British Hypertension Society guidelines and European guidelines (2019) recommend that they are used as first-line agents in patients above the age of 55 and those of African or Caribbean descent. Thiazides are also a first-line alternative agent for this group. CCBs are also recommended as first line in isolated systolic hypertension, patients with left ventricular hypertrophy, and women. They have been shown to reduce long-term cardiovascular risk and are generally well tolerated. There are cautions with co-prescribing with other drugs that affect the cytochrome P450 (CYP) 3A4 system and in patients with left ventricular systolic impairment. Only non-dihydropyridine CCBs should be considered for use in proteinuric nephropathy, preferably in conjunction with an agent that blocks the renin–angiotensin–aldosterone system. Nifedipine is the only calcium antagonist that has been safely tested for use in pregnancy.

Along with ACE inhibitors, CCBs are also recommended for use in patients with diabetes and those with the metabolic syndrome. Meta-analyses also suggest that calcium antagonists have a slightly higher efficacy in stroke prevention and in delaying progression of carotid atherosclerosis, compared to diuretics and beta blockers.

KEY REFERENCES

ALLHAT Collaborative Research Group (2004). Major cardiovascular events in hypertensive patients randomized to doxazosin vs chlorthalidone: the antihypertensive and lipid-lowering treatment to prevent heart attack trial (ALLHAT). *JAMA* **283**:1967–75.

Arnett DK, Blumenthal RS, Albert MA, et al. (2020). 2019 ACC/AHA Guideline on the primary prevention of cardiovascular disease: executive summary: a report of the American College of Cardiology/American Heart Association Task Force on Clinical Practice Guidelines. J Am Coll Cardiol 75:840.

Bakris GL, Weir MR, Secic M, Campbell B, Weis-McNulty A. (2004). Differential effects of calcium antagonist subclasses on markers of nephropathy progression. Kidney Int 65:1991–2002. doi:10.1111/j.1523-1755.2004.00620.x. PMID: 15149313.

Basile J (2004). The role of existing and newer calcium channel blockers in the treatment of hypertension. J Clin Hypertens 6:621–9.

Costanzo P, Perrone-Filardi P, Petretta M, et al. (2009). Calcium channel blockers and cardiovascular outcomes: a meta-analysis of 175,634 patients. J Hypertens 27:1136–51.

Dahlöf B, Sever PS, Poulter NR, et al.; ASCOT Investigators (2005). Prevention of cardiovascular events with an antihypertensive regimen of amlodipine adding perindopril as required versus atenolol adding bendroflumethiazide as required, in the Anglo-Scandinavian Cardiac Outcomes Trial-Blood Pressure Lowering Arm (ASCOT-BPLA): a multicentre randomised controlled trial. Lancet 366:895–906.

Godfraind T (2017). Discovery and development of calcium channel blockers. Front Pharmacol 8:286.

Opie L. (2001). Calcium channel blockers in hypertension: reappraisal after new trials and major meta-analyses. Am J Hypertens 14:1074–81.

Pahor M, Psaty BM, Alderman MH (2000). Health outcomes associated with calcium antagonists compared with other first-line antihypertensive therapies: a meta-analysis of randomised controlled trials. Lancet 356:1949–54.

Rothwell PM, Howard SC, Dolan E, et al. (2010). Effects of beta blockers and calcium-channel blockers on within-individual variability in blood pressure and risk of stroke. Lancet Neurol 9:469–80.

Staessen JA, Wang JG, Thijs L (2002). Calcium-channel blockade and cardiovascular prognosis: recent evidence from clinical outcome trials. Am J Hypertens 15(7 Pt 2):85S–93S.

The Lancet (2019). NICE hypertension guidelines: a pragmatic compromise. Lancet 394:806.

The Task Force for the management of arterial hypertension of the European Society of Hypertension (ESH) and of the European Society of Cardiology (2018). ESH/ESC Guidelines for the management of arterial hypertension. Eur Heart J 39:3021–104.

Wang AL, Iadecola C, Wang G (2017). New generations of dihydropyridines for treatment of hypertension. J Geriatr Cardiol 14:67–72.

CHAPTER 17

Blockers of the renin-angiotensin-aldosterone system in hypertension

Ify R. Mordi and Chim C. Lang

> **KEY POINTS**
>
> * The renin–angiotensin–aldosterone system (RAAS) is an integral part of the body's mechanism for maintaining normal blood volume and pressure, and therefore plays a key role in hypertension.
> * Blockers of the RAAS therefore are potent antihypertensive agents and have been shown to improve blood pressure and improve prognosis.
> * Guidelines recommend their use as first-line agents in the management of hypertension.

17.1 Role of the renin-angiotensin-aldosterone system in hypertension and its associated end-organ damage

The renin–angiotensin–aldosterone system (RAAS) plays a key pathophysiological role in hypertension and this has been discussed in detail in Chapter 2. However, we will discuss some of the salient points in this section. The RAAS plays a critical role in blood pressure (BP) homeostasis and fluid and electrolyte balance, and is a central regulator of cardiovascular and renal function. The activity of the octapeptide hormone angiotensin II is widely targeted clinically in the treatment of hypertension and numerous cardiovascular and kidney diseases. In addition to its peripheral and central effects, angiotensin II can act as a paracrine, autocrine, and intracrine hormone. Angiotensin II exerts its vasoconstrictor effects by binding to angiotensin type 1 receptors (AT-1Rs) in resistance vessels. Angiotensin II also acts in the brain to influence responses that modulate BP, including water intake (via vasopressin secretion) and the sympathetic nervous system. In addition, angiotensin II directly increases sodium and water reabsorption in the kidney and stimulates aldosterone release from the zona glomerulosa of the adrenal gland. There is increasing evidence of the role of a dysregulated RAAS as an important contributor to the pathophysiology of end-organ damage in hypertension, including increases in arterial and cardiac stiffness, left ventricular hypertrophy, abnormalities of cardiac diastolic relaxation, and eventual development of heart failure. Dysregulation of the RAAS is also implicated in the pathogenesis of diabetic nephropathy. The exact role and mechanisms by which an activated RAAS contributes to the development of cardiovascular fibrosis and stiffness are still not clear, but it is likely that abnormalities in sodium homeostasis, endothelial cell/vascular smooth muscle cell dysfunction, and epithelial sodium channel activation of AT-1Rs and mineralocorticoid receptors may be involved in these changes. The pathophysiology is clearly complex as additional risk factors, such as genetic determinants, insulin resistance, diabetes mellitus, obesity, and ageing, are also involved in the development and progression of cardiovascular fibrosis.

Since the discovery of the role of the RAAS in hypertension, several drug classes have been developed to target its various aspects, primarily with the aim of decreasing angiotensin II and aldosterone activity. We will now go on to discuss each of these in turn, with reference to clinical trials that have shown that RAAS blockade can contribute to prevention of cardiovascular and renal disease in hypertension.

17.2 Angiotensin-converting enzyme inhibitors

Angiotensin-converting enzyme inhibitors (ACEIs) are perhaps the most widely studied RAAS blockers used for treatment of hypertension and are first-line antihypertensives in most treatment guidelines. ACEIs act by stopping the conversion of angiotensin I to angiotensin II by angiotensin-converting enzyme (ACE). Decreased production of angiotensin II increases natriuresis and lowers BP by vasodilatory action. They also reduce breakdown of bradykinin, which again leads to further vasodilatation. The initial BP-lowering response is greater in patients with high plasma renin activity. However, their long-term antihypertensive effect is not related to plasma renin activity.

Overall, ACEIs have consistently been shown to reduce BP, although the reduction may be more modest when compared to other antihypertensive drug classes. In the ALLHAT trial, the systolic BP (SBP) was significantly higher at 5 years in patients randomized to lisinopril, compared to those randomized to chlorthalidone (2 mmHg). Whilst the reduction in BP may be more modest when compared to other antihypertensives, overall in ACEI trials on hypertension, there has been a consistent reduction in all-cause mortality (around 5% relative risk reduction).

ACEIs seem to be less effective in individuals of black African/Caribbean origin, in particular males. This is thought to be because black individuals have low renin levels, although the mechanisms are not completely understood. Given the prevalence of hypertension in black patients, this is an important consideration. Most guidelines recommend that calcium channel blockers and thiazide-like diuretics are used as first-line antihypertensive treatments in black patients, with angiotensin receptor blockers (ARBs) preferred in combination therapy, though ACEIs can still be used. Black patients can achieve the same levels of BP reduction with combination therapy as other ethnic groups and still derive the equivalent benefit from BP lowering; thus, it is vital that they are well treated and they may need higher doses of ACEIs (or ARBs).

ACEIs also have good evidence for reducing end-organ damage. ACEIs reduce albuminuria more than other antihypertensive drug classes and reduce the risk of end-stage renal disease. ACEIs also cause regression of left ventricular hypertrophy, not only via their BP-lowering effects, but also by other mechanisms such as reduction of angiotensin II (which promotes myocyte growth, independent of loading conditions). Finally, ACEIs have also been shown to delay progression to macroalbuminuria in patients with type 2 diabetes and hypertension.

Other considerations for ACEIs are that they are contraindicated in patients with bilateral renal artery stenosis due to the risk of acute renal failure, and that they are associated with a risk of angio-oedema due to prevention of breakdown of bradykinin. Angio-oedema occurs more frequently in females and black individuals, though the overall incidence is between 0.1% and 0.7%.

Overall, ACEIs are one of the cornerstones of antihypertensive therapy and are recommended as first line in all clinical guidelines. They are also useful in patients with concomitant conditions such as heart failure, myocardial infarction, type 2 diabetes, and renal disease, and so retain a key position in treatment in hypertension.

17.3 Angiotensin receptor blockers

ARBs are commonly thought of as alternatives to ACEIs in patients who cannot tolerate ACEIs (predominantly due to cough). Nevertheless, they appear to be at least as efficacious as ACEIs for BP lowering and reductions in major adverse cardiovascular outcomes. The first large study in patients with hypertension was the Losartan Intervention for Endpoint reduction in hypertension (LIFE) study, a randomized controlled trial involving patients with hypertension and left ventricular hypertrophy. The trial showed that losartan prevented more cardiovascular morbidity and death than the comparator atenolol for a similar reduction in BP. Overall, meta-analyses of clinical trial data show that ARBs and ACEIs have similar BP-lowering efficacy (approximately $-8/-5$ mmHg) and similar reductions in death, cardiovascular events, or cardiovascular death. In the Ongoing Telmisartan Alone and in Combination With Ramipril Global Endpoint Trial (ONTARGET) trial, there was no difference in incidence of cardiovascular outcomes between ramipril and telmisartan in patients at high cardiovascular risk, though only around 70% of participants had a history of hypertension. ARBs also have other beneficial cardiovascular and renal effects, with reductions in left ventricular mass and proteinuria, similar to ACEIs.

There is consistent evidence showing that ARBs are better tolerated than ACEIs, with cough being the most consistent side effect associated with ACEIs. In a meta-analysis including 198,130 patients, the incidence of cough with ACEIs was 11.48%, with a withdrawal rate of 2.57%. Withdrawal rates with ARBs are around 22% lower than with ACEIs. In fact, discontinuation rates for ARBs are equivalent to placebo in clinical trials, reflecting their high tolerability. Combined with the risk of angio-oedema with ACEIs, there is certainly an argument that ARBs might be considered a reasonable alternative to ACEIs and, indeed some would argue, should be considered as first-line RAAS blockers for hypertension. Similarly to ACEIs, ARBs should be avoided in individuals with bilateral renal artery stenosis.

For a long time, it was hypothesized that there might be benefits to dual RAAS blockade with ACEIs and ARBs, and indeed for a time, this was in several guidelines. Despite this, dual blockade failed to provide additive BP-lowering effects and, in fact, caused a substantially higher number of renal adverse events. As a consequence, combined use of ACEIs and ARBs is not recommended and indeed contraindicated in any current hypertension guideline.

17.4 Mineralocorticoid receptor antagonists

The first strong evidence suggesting that spironolactone might be useful in resistant hypertension was from the Anglo-Scandinavian Cardiac Outcomes Trial-Blood Pressure Lowering Arm (ASCOT-BPLA) study. In this trial, which compared two open-label antihypertensive regimens for prevention of coronary heart disease events in hypertensive patients with additional cardiovascular risk factors, but no history of coronary heart disease, spironolactone was most commonly used as a fourth-line add-on therapy for hypertension. In a subsequent post hoc analysis of this trial, spironolactone use was associated with significant BP reductions at 1.2 years (systolic -21.9 mmHg; diastolic -9.5 mmHg) in 1411 patients already taking a mean of 29 antihypertensive drugs. Spironolactone use was associated with significant increases in potassium and creatinine levels.

This hypothesis-generating finding was tested in the Prevention and Treatment of Hypertension With Algorithm based Therapy-2 trial (PATHWAY-2) trial. In this double-blind, placebo-controlled crossover trial, spironolactone (25–50 mg once daily) was compared to bisoprolol, doxazosin, and placebo in patients with office SBP readings $\geq$140 mmHg (or $\geq$135 mmHg for patients with diabetes) and home SBP readings $\geq$130 mmHg despite being on three antihypertensives (maximal tolerated doses of ACEI/ARB, calcium channel blocker, and diuretic). Spironolactone caused a significant reduction in home SBP, compared to placebo (-8.70 mmHg; 95% confidence interval (CI) -9.72 to -7.69), doxazosin (-4.03 mmHg; 95% CI -5.04 to -3.02), and bisoprolol (-4.48 mmHg; 95% CI -5.50 to -3.46), with no significant increase in adverse events, compared to both active comparators. These results were replicated in a smaller trial of patients with resistant hypertension and type 2 diabetes where spironolactone caused a significant reduction in BP and urine albumin:creatinine ratio after 16 weeks.

Eplerenone is a more selective mineralocorticoid receptor antagonist (MRA) than spironolactone, with less anti-androgen effects, albeit with slightly weaker cardiovascular effects and, at present, higher cost. There are no direct head-to-head data to compare the two. However, eplerenone may be a reasonable alternative for treatment of hypertension in patients who are unable to tolerate spironolactone for reasons such as gynaecomastia. Eplerenone also reduces BP in patients with uncontrolled/resistant hypertension.

There are few specific data on major cardiovascular outcomes with use of MRAs in hypertension. Overall, these results support the use of spironolactone as an add-on therapy for patients with difficult-to-control hypertension. They are also useful in treatment of hypertension associated with primary hyperaldosteronism and in patients with heart failure.

Recently, non-steroidal MRAs have been developed. These have the advantage of being selective for mineralocorticoid receptors, rather than glucocorticoid or sex hormone receptors. The first in this class is finerenone. Esaxerenone, another non-steroidal MRA, has been shown to reduce BP in hypertensive patients, similarly to eplerenone, and is approved for use in Japan. There are few long-term data specifically in patients with hypertension. However, finerenone did cause a significant reduction in urine albumin:creatinine ratio and slower decline in renal function, compared to placebo, at 36 months in patients with chronic kidney disease and diabetes in the The Finerenone in Reducing Kidney Failure and Disease Progression in Diabetic Kidney Disease trial (FIDELIO-DKD) trial; 97% of patients in the trial had a history of hypertension, with a mean blood pressure of 138/76 mmHg. Blood pressure change was modest with finerenone versus placebo (−2.58 versus −0.12 mmHg at 36 months). Patients in the finerenone group had a significantly reduced incidence of primary renal outcomes (renal failure, sustained estimated glomerular filtration rate (eGFR) decrease, or renal death), as well as a reduced likelihood of major adverse cardiovascular events. The more selective nature of non-steroidal MRAs, a reduced incidence of hyperkalaemia, and a safer renal profile make this class of MRAs attractive for further use in hypertension.

17.5 Angiotensin receptor-neprilysin inhibitors

Neprilysin is an endopeptidase which (primarily) breaks down natriuretic peptides. Thus, inhibition of neprilysin should increase endogenous natriuretic peptide levels and prevent degradation of vasoactive peptides such as bradykinin, and adrenomedullin, leading to natriuresis and vasodilatation, both potentially reducing BP. Initial attempts to combine RAAS blockade with neprilysin inhibition used ACEIs (omapatrilat) and did demonstrate a significant reduction in BP, compared to enalapril. However, this was complicated by an unacceptable increase in the risk of angio-oedema due to dual inhibition of bradykinin breakdown (as well as substance P and neurokinin), which led to its use being abandoned.

This did, however, lead to the idea of combining neprilysin inhibition with an ARB. In theory, ARBs do not inhibit breakdown of bradykinin and so should have lower risk of angio-oedema. At present, sacubitril/valsartan is the only angiotensin receptor–neprilysin inhibitor (ARNI) available for clinical use and was originally developed for use in patients with heart failure. There is evidence that sacubitril/valsartan may have greater efficacy in hypertension than ACEIs/ARBs in studies of shorter duration. In a study of 1328 adults with 'mild to moderate hypertension' (mean sitting diastolic BP of 90–109 mmHg after antihypertensive washout, or 95–109 mmHg for untreated patients), sacubitril/valsartan caused a significant reduction in SBP, compared to valsartan (approximately 3 mmHg), at 8 weeks. In the Prospective Comparison of Angiotensin Receptor Neprilysin Inhibitor With Angiotensin Receptor Blocker Measuring Arterial Stiffness in the Elderly (PARAMETER) study, sacubitril/valsartan caused a 3.7 mmHg lower SBP, central aortic blood BP, and pulse pressure, compared to olmesartan, at 12 weeks in older patients (>60 years) with hypertension, though there was no change in aortic pulse wave velocity. Overall, in a meta-analysis of 11 randomized controlled trials including 6028 patients with hypertension, sacubitril/valsartan caused significant reductions in SBP and diastolic BP, compared to either active comparator (usually ARB) or placebo, with no significant increase in adverse events, even at the highest dose. Compared with ARBs, 200 mg of sacubitril/valsartan reduced SBP and diastolic BP by 4.62 mmHg and 2.13 mmHg, respectively, whereas 400 mg of sacubitril/valsartan reduced SBP and diastolic BP by 5.50 mmHg and 2.51 mmHg. Importantly, as predicted, no significant increase in angio-oedema has been noted with sacubitril/valsartan in any studies.

There are little long-term data to confirm whether the additional reduction in BP with sacubitril/valsartan translates to improved cardiovascular outcome in patients with hypertension, with no dedicated outcome studies published as yet. Some data suggesting this are available from large heart failure outcome trials. In the pivotal phase III outcome trial in patients with heart failure with reduced ejection fraction Prospective comparison of Angiotensin Receptor-neprilysin inhibitor (ARNI) with Angiotensin converting enzyme inhibitor (ACEI) to Determine Impact on Global Mortality and morbidity in Heart Failure (PARADIGM-HF), sacubitril/valsartan caused a 4–6 mmHg reduction in SBP, compared to enalapril, at 4 months, and hypotensive events were more common in those in the sacubitril/valsartan arm (although treatment discontinuation rates were similar and the benefit of sacubitril/valsartan over enalapril was consistent, regardless of BP). In PARADIGM-HF, the benefit of sacubitril/valsartan over enalapril was consistent, regardless of aetiology, including in those with hypertensive heart failure. In Prospective Comparison of ARNI with ARB Global Outcomes in HF with Preserved Ejection Fraction (PARAGON-HF) (sacubitril/valsartan versus enalapril in patients with heart failure with preserved ejection fraction), the nominal non-significant reduction in the primary outcomes of mortality and heart failure hospitalization was independent of the BP-lowering effect, though again sacubitril/valsartan did cause a lower BP over the trial.

As yet, sacubitril/valsartan is not a standard treatment for hypertension and should never be prescribed in combination with ACEIs due to the risk of angio-oedema. Nevertheless, it does have a significant additional antihypertensive effect over other ACEI/ARBs, and as we gain more clinical experience with ARNIs, its use may become more commonplace in patients with hypertension.

17.6 Direct renin inhibitors

Theoretically, it was logical to presume that blockade of the RAAS in the first step (conversion of angiotensinogen to angiotensin I by renin) would perhaps lead to more complete control of the RAAS and incremental benefit over ACEIs and ARBs by reducing renin activity. Only one direct renin inhibitor has been developed—aliskiren. In early trials of short duration, aliskiren demonstrated marked reductions in SBP and diastolic BP, compared to placebo (>10 mmHg by 8 weeks at maximum dosage), and similar reductions compared to ACEIs. Given the similar efficacy in BP reduction, compared to ACEIs, however, the role of aliskiren as an antihypertensive remained unclear. A recent meta-analysis of data from these short-term trials showed that aliskiren was not associated with a significantly different effect on mortality or myocardial infarction, compared to ACEIs. However, long-term data were lacking.

Given the presumed benefit of suppression of plasma renin activity (which is increased when ACEIs/ARBs are used), it was also thought that more complete RAAS blockade with aliskiren in combination with ACEIs or ARBs might also lead to improved outcome. This combination, however, caused a significantly increased risk of hyperkalaemia, compared to monotherapy with either drug (hazard ratio for hyperkalaemia with combination therapy 1.58 (95% CI 1.24–2.02) versus ACEI/ARB; 1.67 (95% CI 1.01–2.79) versus aliskiren). Indeed, combination therapy with aliskiren and ACEIs/ARBs was evaluated in the The Aliskiren *Trial* in Type 2 Diabetes Using Cardiorenal Endpoints (ALTITUDE) trial, which was stopped prematurely due to a significant increase in adverse events leading to discontinuation of aliskiren (predominantly hyperkalaemia and hypotension) without any evidence of efficacy.

The results of this trial, in combination with other data showing no significant additional benefit over ACEIs/ARBs, have meant that presently aliskiren is not commonly used in management of hypertension, and its use in combination with ACEIs/ARBs not currently recommended in the most recent European or American hypertension guidelines.

17.7 The place of RAAS blockers in clinical management of hypertension

Current guideline recommendations for use of RAAS blockers in hypertension are summarized in Table 17.1.

ACEIs/ARBs are broadly interchangeable in guidelines and are uniformly recommended as first-line therapy alone or in combination with calcium channel blockers or thiazide-like diuretics. Some caveats are made, specifically in older patients and those of black African or Caribbean origin, in whom ARBs might specifically be preferred. Spironolactone is also generally accepted as the first additional treatment which should be used in patients with resistant hypertension (other MRAs are not mentioned in the guidelines, reflecting the limited evidence

Table 17.1 Summary of international clinical practice guideline recommendations for RAAS blockers in management of hypertension

	NICE (UK) 2019	European Society of Cardiology (2018)	ACC/AHA (2017)	ISH (2020)
ACEI/ARB	First-line antihypertensive in all patients with type 2 diabetes or in those without type 2 diabetes aged <55 years and not of black African/Caribbean origin	First line in combination with CCB or thiazide-like diuretic	First-line antihypertensive. Use ARB in patients with a history of angio-oedema	First-line therapy in combination with CCB or thiazide-like diuretic
MRA	Consider low-dose spironolactone in 'step 4' for patients with resistant hypertension who have a blood potassium level of ≤4.5 mmol/L	Add spironolactone 25–50 mg for patients with resistant hypertension on ACEI/ARB + CCB + thiazide	Preferred agents as add-on therapy in resistant hypertension and primary hyperaldosteronism	Use spironolactone in resistant hypertension ('step 4' after combination therapy with ACEI/ARB + CCB + thiazide)
ARNI	Not mentioned	Can be used in patients with HFrEF as an alternative to ACEI/ARB	Not mentioned	Indicated in patients with HFrEF (for HF, rather than hypertension per se)
Direct renin inhibitor	Not mentioned	Not included in treatment algorithm	Do not use in combination with ACEI/ARB	Not mentioned

NICE, National Institute for Health and Care Excellence; ACC, American College of Cardiology; AHA, American Heart Association; ISH, International Society of Hypertension; ACEI, angiotensin-converting enzyme inhibitor; ARB, angiotensin receptor blocker; CCB, calcium channel blocker; MRA, mineralocorticoid receptor antagonist; ARNI, angiotensin receptor–neprilysin inhibitor; HFrEF, heart failure with reduced ejection fraction; HF, heart failure.

for their use in hypertension). Sacubitril/valsartan is briefly mentioned and has a role in patients with heart failure with reduced ejection fraction and concomitant hypertension, in whom the benefits on all-cause mortality and heart failure hospitalization over ACEIs might make it the preferred choice. Aliskiren has fallen out of favour in recent times, and guidelines generally make little mention of it (if at all), reflecting its rare use in current clinical practice.

17.8 Conclusion

In conclusion, blockade of the RAAS plays a key role in the management of hypertension. In particular, ACEIs and ARBs should be considered first-line therapy in the majority of patients with hypertension, and indeed there may be particularly compelling indications for their use (type 2 diabetes, heart failure, prior myocardial infarction). Recent data also support the use of MRAs in treatment of resistant hypertension. There are an abundance of data and clinical experience to show that ACEIs and ARBs also improve cardiovascular outcomes, in addition to their BP-lowering effects, and this class of drugs continue to play an important role in the management of hypertension.

KEY REFERENCES

Matchar DB, McCrory DC, Orlando LA, et al. (2008). Systematic review: comparative effectiveness of angiotensin-converting enzyme inhibitors and angiotensin II receptor blockers for treating essential hypertension. Ann Intern Med 148:16–29.

Schmieder RE, Hilgers KF, Schlaich MP, Schmidt BM (2007). Renin–angiotensin system and cardiovascular risk. Lancet 369:1208–19.

Te Riet L, van Esch JH, Roks AJ, van den Meiracker AH, Danser AH (2015). Hypertension: renin–angiotensin–aldosterone system alterations. Circ Res 116:960–75.

van Vark LC, Bertrand M, Akkerhuis KM, et al. (2012). Angiotensin-converting enzyme inhibitors reduce mortality in hypertension: a meta-analysis of randomized clinical trials of renin–angiotensin–aldosterone system inhibitors involving 158,998 patients. Eur Heart J 33:2088–97.

Weir MR, Dzau VJ (1999). The renin–angiotensin–aldosterone system: a specific target for hypertension management. Am J Hypertens 12:205S–13S.

CHAPTER 18

Other antihypertensive agents

Shankar Patil, Muzahir Tayebjee, and Sunil K. Nadar

KEY POINTS

- Drugs such as alpha adrenergic blockers, centrally acting drugs, and direct vasodilators are used as add-on therapy in resistant hypertension.
- These agents are not recommended for initial therapy due to lack of evidence for long-term prognostic benefit and their side effects.
- Alpha adrenergic blockers, such as doxazosin, may be used in patients with benign prostatic hypertrophy.
- Alpha methyldopa is used predominantly in pregnancy-related hypertension.
- There are many new agents currently being investigated for management of hypertension. These target different pathways of the renin–angiotensin–aldosterone system and the brain renin–angiotensin system.

18.1 Introduction

Apart from the first-line agents calcium channel blockers, diuretics, angiotensin-converting enzyme (ACE) inhibitors, and beta blockers, there are other agents, such as alpha adrenoreceptor antagonists, centrally acting agents, vasodilators, and aldosterone receptor antagonists, that have roles in the management of hypertension. These agents generally do not have significant evidence of long-term prognostic benefit in the management of hypertension, as seen with first-line agents. In addition, they are often not as well tolerated as first-line agents. The various international guidelines on management of hypertension therefore typically reserve these agents for the management of resistant hypertension, patients who are intolerant to first-line agents, and specific subgroups of hypertensive patients. This chapter covers the pharmacology and indications for these agents. This chapter will also focus on some of the novel agents that are undergoing clinical trials which could be part of our management protocols in the future.

18.2 Alpha adrenoreceptor antagonists (alpha blockers)

Alpha adrenoreceptors ($\alpha 1$ and $\alpha 2$) are widely distributed on vascular smooth muscle cells. $\alpha 1$ receptors predominantly mediate vasoconstriction, and blocking them results in non-specific arterial and venous dilatation and consequent blood pressure (BP) reduction.

There are two types of alpha blockers:

- Selective alpha blockers (prazosin, doxazosin, terazosin) can be used as add-on therapy for uncontrolled hypertension and benign prostatic hypertrophy.
- Non-selective alpha blockers (phenoxybenzamine, phentolamine) are used to treat hypertensive crisis associated with proven phaeochromocytoma.

Main side effects are dizziness, orthostatic hypotension, nasal congestion, somnolence, headache, and reflex tachycardia. Doxazosin and prazosin tend to cause fluid retention and should be avoided in heart failure. These medications can complicate cataract surgery by inducing sudden iris prolapse and pupil constriction during surgery—also known as intraoperative floppy iris syndrome. They can also cause priapism. Phenoxybenzamine and phentolamine are contraindicated in breastfeeding mothers. Elderly patients are particularly prone to orthostatic hypotension and female patients are likely to experience urinary stress incontinence. Patients on phosphodiesterase-5 inhibitors (sildenafil, tadalafil) should avoid alpha blockers as this may result in profound hypotension.

When used as first line of treatment for hypertension, patients had a higher risk of cardiovascular events in two major clinical trials (Antihypertensive and Lipid-Lowering Treatment to Prevent Heart Attack Trial (ALLHAT) and Veterans Administration Study). Guidelines from the National Institute for Health and Care Excellence (NICE) and recent American and European guidelines on management of hypertension recommend using alpha blockers with other antihypertensive drugs in treatment-resistant hypertension. Table 18.1 summarizes commonly used drugs from this group and their typical doses and pharmacokinetics.

18.3 Centrally acting agents

Central BP regulation is mediated via alpha adrenoreceptors located in the pons and medulla. Centrally acting agents cross the blood–brain barrier and act on post-synaptic $\alpha 2$ receptors, reducing brainstem sympathetic outflow and thereby causing peripheral vasodilatation and lowering BP. They include alpha methyldopa and imidazolidine-related compounds such as clonidine and moxonidine.

Alpha methyldopa was one of the most widely used antihypertensive agents a few decades ago. However, due to side effects and the prognostic benefit demonstrated by other agents, its use has been restricted to pregnancy-related hypertension and resistant hypertension. It is still widely used in some countries due to its low cost. It is converted to methyl noradrenaline centrally to decrease the adrenergic outflow by alpha-2 agonistic action from the central nervous system, leading to reduced total peripheral resistance and decreased systemic BP.

Table 18.1 Commonly used alpha adrenergic blockers

Drug	Dose and administration	Comments	Pharmacokinetics
Doxazosin	Oral: 1–16 mg/day once daily	Can also be used for benign prostatic hypertrophy. Use with caution in patients with heart failure as it can cause fluid retention	Rapidly absorbed orally. Plasma elimination is biphasic, with a terminal elimination half-life of 22 hours. Metabolized extensively in the liver
Prazosin	Oral: 6–20 mg/day in divided doses	As above; occasionally used for post-traumatic stress disorder	Good oral absorption, with peak levels noted 1–3 hours after administration. Extensively metabolized in the liver. High binding to plasma proteins
Phenoxybenzamine	Oral: starting dose 10 mg/day to a maximum of 1–2 mg/kg/day in two divided doses	May need concomitant use of a beta blocker to control resultant tachycardia	Variable oral absorption, with bioavailability of 20–30%. Half-life of 24 hours and extensively metabolized in the liver
Phentolamine	Intravenous: 1–5 mg bolus and 6–40 mg/hour, titrating according to BP	Usually used for hypertensive emergencies such as catecholamine storm during phaeochromocytoma surgery	Peak action at 10–20 minutes after intravenous administration. Half-life of 19 minutes and metabolized in the liver

Clonidine is a centrally acting alpha agonist agent. It is recommended for use mainly in cases of resistant hypertension. In addition to hypertension, it is also used for managing symptoms of drug withdrawal and improving symptoms of attention-deficit/hyperactivity disorder in some patients, and treating some psychiatric illnesses such as stress, sleep disorders, and post-traumatic stress disorder. It is also a mild sedative and can be used in restless legs syndrome and migraine.

Moxonidine is a second-generation, centrally acting antihypertensive drug. It is an α2/I1-imidazoline receptor agonist in the rostroventrolateral medulla, thereby reducing the activity of the sympathetic nervous system. It has more affinity for the I1-imidazoline receptor than for the α2 receptor, in contrast to clonidine which has almost similar affinity to both receptors. In addition, moxonidine also demonstrates favourable effects on parameters of the insulin resistance syndrome, such as improved insulin resistance and glucose tolerance and also increased sodium excretion. It has also been shown to release growth hormone. Current guidelines recommend using moxonidine for mild to moderate essential hypertension and as an add-on in patients with resistant hypertension.

The main side effects of these centrally acting agents are postural hypotension, bradycardia, dry mouth, sexual impotence, haemolytic anaemia (positive Coombs' test), extrapyramidal disorders, hepatitis, sedation, withdrawal phenomenon, and tolerance. The dosages and administration and pharmacokinetics of these drugs are summarized in Table 18.2.

Table 18.2 Commonly used centrally acting agents

Drug	Dose and administration	Pharmacokinetics
Alpha methyldopa	Maintenance: oral 500 mg to 2 g/day, in divided doses, up to a maximum of 3 g/day. Hypertensive emergency: 250–500 mg intravenously over 30–60 minutes every 6 hours, up to a maximum of 1 g every 6 hours or 4 g/day; change to oral as above once BP controlled	Used mainly for pregnancy-related hypertension and hypertensive emergencies. Bioavailability after oral administration is incomplete at around 25% at 2 hours and around 50% at 4 hours. It is weakly protein-binding and, being lipid-soluble, easily crosses the blood–brain barrier. Peak effect is at 4–6 hours after oral administration; 70% of the drug is excreted in the urine and the rest is excreted unchanged in the faeces. Dose may need adjusting in renal failure
Clonidine	Oral: 0.2–0.6 mg daily, up to a maximum of 2.4 mg daily in divided doses	Rapidly absorbed orally. BP starts falling within an hour of ingestion. Peak effect within 2–4 hours. Elimination half-life is 12–16 hours. Around 50% is excreted unchanged in the urine and 50% is metabolized in the liver. Excreted primarily by the kidneys, and so the dose may have to be adjusted in renal failure
Moxonidine	Oral: 0.2–0.6 mg once daily	Rapid and almost complete absorption after oral administration. Peak levels in plasma are noted almost 1 hour after administration. Plasma half-life is around 2 hours. Excreted by the kidney, and so the dose has to be adjusted in renal failure

18.4 Direct vasodilators

This group of drugs includes agents such as nitrates, nitroprusside, and hydralazine. Nitrates and nitroprusside act directly on the vascular endothelium via nitric oxide release, which stimulates cyclic guanosine monophosphate (cGMP)-mediated vascular smooth muscle relaxation and vasodilatation. Hydralazine, on the other hand, also acts directly on vascular smooth muscle and induces arteriolar vaso-dilatation by preventing oxidation of nitric oxide and thereby lowering BP.

These agents are not used for routine management of hypertension but are predominantly used in hypertensive emergencies where BP needs to be reduced urgently. Main side effects include headache, cutaneous flushing, hypotension, tachycardia, and angina. Prolonged sodium nitroprusside use can cause thio-cyanate toxicity.

When used alone, they can stimulate baroreceptors, leading to reflex tachy-cardia, a rise in cardiac output, and increased cardiac contraction. This can trigger angina. Hence, they should be combined with beta adrenergic blockers.

Minoxidil is another direct vasodilator that acts on adenosine triphosphate (ATP)-sensitive potassium channels on vascular smooth muscle, causing arterial dilatation. However, its use is associated with activation of the sympathetic ner-vous system and an increase in plasma renin activity, which over time offsets any benefit of BP lowering with the vasodilatory effect. Its use now is restricted mainly to patients who are not responsive to other medications and where intolerance restricts the use of other drugs. However, it is used extensively as a topical prep-aration for male pattern baldness.

18.5 Novel antihypertensive drugs in development

In addition to the antihypertensive agents mentioned above, there are many agents that are in various stages of research. We have listed a few of the im-portant ones below.

18.5.1 Centrally acting aminopeptidase A inhibitors

Various experimental animal models have not only proven the existence of a functional renin–angiotensin system (RAS) in the brain, but also shown hyper-activity of brain aminopeptidase A (APA) to be responsible for the development and maintenance of hypertension. Targeting brain APA activity has been shown to decrease BP. Firibastat, previously named QGC001 or RB150, is the first orally active, specific, and selective inhibitor of brain APA. It is a prodrug that is cleaved by brain reductases on entry into the brain to active molecules called EC33, which, in turn, inhibit brain APA activity, block brain angiotensin III generation, and decrease BP. A phase II, open-label, multicentric dose-titrating study showed firibastat to be effective in lowering BP in a high-risk population. A phase III study Firibastat in Treatment-resistant Hypertension (FRESH) has currently finsished recruiting at the end of 2021 and the results should be out by 2022.

18.5.2 Aldosterone synthase inhibitors

Targeting aldosterone synthesis to prevent the deleterious effects of angiotensin II has resulted in research on novel agents for resistant hypertension. The reactive increase in aldosterone levels as a result of inhibiting the aldosterone receptor could be counteracted by aldosterone synthase inhibitors. Fadrozole was the first aldosterone synthase inhibitor to be trialled in humans, but lack of significant efficacy led to its discontinuation. LCI 699 is the first aldosterone synthase inhibitor to progress to phase II trials, with these studies showing good pressure-lowering effect (-7.1 mmHg) with a dose of 1 mg twice daily, compared to placebo. It does not prevent adverse effects such as sodium retention and potassium excretion mediated by aldosterone and its effect was not shown to superior to that of eplerenone. Hence, there is a search for aldosterone synthase inhibitors with greater specificity. Multiple phase I trials involving next-generation aldosterone synthase inhibitors with greater selectivity against cortisol synthase, which is an enzyme closely related to aldosterone synthase, have been reported in humans, with promising results. More data are awaited before these agents can move on to phase II trials.

18.5.3 Natriuretic peptide receptor agonists

Atrial natriuretic peptide (ANP) and brain natriuretic peptide (BNP) refer to peptides that induce natriuresis and vasodilatation. ANP is produced in response to atrial myocyte stretch and acts on ANP receptors in renal, vascular, and cardiac tissues. Their major role is to counteract the vasopressor effects of aldosterone.

PL3994, a natriuretic peptide receptor agonist (NPRA), has shown BP-lowering effect and natriuresis in healthy volunteers in phase I trials. In phase IIa clinical trials, combining PL3994 with ACE inhibitors produced a pronounced BP reduction, suggesting a synergistic effect. The main drawback is that ANP agonists cannot be administered orally, but via a subcutaneous injection. Although it has been shown to reduce BP, it is currently undergoing trials primarily as a treatment for heart failure.

18.5.4 Soluble epoxide hydrolase inhibitors

Soluble epoxide hydrolase (sEH) is an enzyme expressed in various tissues, including liver and vascular endothelium. It hydrolyses endogenous lipid epoxides, preventing them from exerting their vasodilatory effects. Inhibiting sEH causes vasodilatation and lowers BP, improves insulin sensitivity, and decreases inflammation.

AR9821 is the first sEH inhibitor that is being investigated in clinical trials. In animal models, it lowered BP, improved vascular function, and reduced renal damage in rats with angiotensin II-induced hypertension. However, a phase I clinical trial in healthy volunteers failed to show any BP-lowering effect. In a separate study, it lowered the activity of sHE in patients with hypertension and diabetes, indicating a possible role in this specific group of patients. It is currently being investigated for its use in heart failure.

18.5.5 Vasopeptidase inhibitors

Vasopeptidase inhibitors are a class of drugs that have dual inhibitory effects on two key enzymes involved in the metabolism of vasoactive peptides. Essentially, they inhibit ACE, thereby blocking the generation of angiotensin II (Ang II); at the same time, they prevent the breakdown of natriuretic peptides by the enzyme neutral endopeptidase. Omapatrilat was the first agent from this class to be investigated in hypertension. It demonstrated a significant BP-lowering effect; however, it was not granted approval due to a high incidence of angio-oedema. As here the breakdown of bradykinins is dually inhibited, the incidence of angio-oedema is much higher than that with ACE inhibitors. This generally halted the trials involving this group of drugs. This, however, gave rise to the concept of using a neprilysin inhibitor separately with an angiotensin receptor blocker—the sacubitril/valsartan combination, which is currently used in the management of heart failure, but also has significant BP-lowering effect.

18.5.6 Sodium–glucose co-transporter-2 inhibitors

This class of drugs (which includes agents such as canagliflozin, dapagliflozin, empagliflozin, and ertugliflozin) are primarily used in the management of diabetes but have been shown to be effective in managing heart failure and lowering BP. They have been shown to improve cardiovascular and renal outcomes possibly by their role in improving blood sugar and BP control. By acting via the sodium–glucose co-transporter (SGLT) system in the kidneys, these drugs cause increased renal glucose excretion, volume contraction, and weight loss, thereby leading to improved BP control and improved cardiovascular events.

Studies on diabetic patients have demonstrated a systolic BP reduction of around 5–12 mmHg, depending on the drug and dose used. However, these were not hypertension trials, and further studies on their use primarily as an antihypertensive agent are lacking.

18.5.7 Non-steroidal mineralocorticoid receptor antagonists

Finerenone is the first in class non-steroidal mineralocorticoid receptor antagonist (MRA) and differs from spironolactone and eplerenone which are steroidal MRAs. It has been shown to have more affinity for the mineralocorticoid receptor than steroidal blockers. Being non-steroidal, it does not have much effect on other receptors such as glucocorticoid and androgen receptors, and therefore has fewer side effects such as gynaecomastia. Preliminary human phase II trials have shown encouraging results, with improvement in BP and cardiovascular outcomes. There are currently two large phase III trials under way in patients with chronic kidney disease and diabetes.

18.5.8 Endothelin receptor antagonists

Endothelins are a family of peptides that are responsible for maintenance of vascular tone; therefore, blocking the receptors on which they act leads to vasodilatation, and hence lowering BP. Atrasentan, avosentan, bosentan, darusentan, and tezosentan are some of the new agents of this class of drugs. A recent meta-analysis of their use in hypertension revealed that on average, all these agents reduced 24-hour BP by 7.65/5.92 mmHg, compared to placebo, but were associated with more side effects than placebo. Aprocitentan, a newer drug of this class, has also shown promising BP-lowering effect in a phase II study. Larger phase III trial data are awaited.

18.5.9 Newer therapeutic targets

There is a considerable amount of interest and research directed towards finding new targets for hypertension treatment that can improve cardiovascular outcomes.

Some of these include:

1. Angiotensin (1-7) analogues
2. Recombinant human ACE 2
3. Ang (1-7) mimetics/Mas receptor agonists
4. Angiotensin (1-7) derivative alamandine
5. Vasoactive intestinal peptide receptor agonists
6. Intestinal Na^+/H^+ exchanger 3 inhibitors
7. Dual L-type calcium channel blockers/endothelin A/B_2 receptor antagonists
8. Ouabain inhibitors
9. Antihypertensive vaccines.

Most of the above potential agents are studied in animal models, with some of them being considered for human phase I trials.

KEY REFERENCES

Anandan SK, Webb HK, Chen D, et al. (2011). 1-(1-acetyl-piperidin-4-yl)-3-adamantan-1-yl-urea (AR9281) as a potent, selective, and orally available soluble epoxide hydrolase inhibitor with efficacy in rodent models of hypertension and dysglycemia. *Bioorg Med Chem Lett* **21**:983–8.

Calhoun DA, White WB, Krum H, et al. (2011). Effects of a novel aldosterone synthase inhibitor for treatment of primary hypertension: results of a randomized, double-blind, placebo- and active-controlled phase 2 trial. *Circulation* **124**:1945–55.

Campbell DJ (2003). Vasopeptidase inhibition: a double-edged sword? *Hypertension* **41**:383–9.

Chen D, Whitcomb R, MacIntyre E, et al. (2012). Pharmacokinetics and pharmacodynamics of AR9281, an inhibitor of soluble epoxide hydrolase, in single- and multiple-dose studies in healthy human subjects. *J Clin Pharmacol* **52**:319–28.

Chen Y, Meng L, Shao H, et al. (2013). Aliskiren vs. other antihypertensive drugs in the treatment of hypertension: a meta-analysis. *Hypertens Res* **36**:252–61.

Chrysant SG, Chrysant GS (2020). New and emerging cardiovascular and antihypertensive drugs. *Expert Opin Drug Saf* **19**:1315–27. doi:10.1080/14740338.2020.1810232

Firibastat in Treatment-resistant Hypertension (FRESH). (2020). A phase 3, double-blind, placebo-controlled, efficacy and safety study of firibastat (QGC001) administered orally, twice daily, over 12 weeks in difficult-to-treat/resistant hypertensive subjects. Available from: https://clinicaltrials.gov/show/NCT04277884

Fournie-Zaluski MC, Fassot C, Valentin B, et al. (2004). Brain renin–angiotensin system blockade by systemically active aminopeptidase A inhibitors: a potential treatment of salt-dependent hypertension. *Proc Natl Acad Sci U S A* **101**:7775–80.

Imig JD (2009). Adenosine 2A receptors and epoxyeicosatrienoic acids: a recipe for salt and blood pressure regulation. *Hypertension* **54**:1223–5.

Jordan R, Stark J, Huskey S, et al. (2008). Phase 1 study of the novel A-type natriuretic receptor agonist, PL-3994, in healthy volunteers. *Journal of Cardiac Failure* **14**(6 suppl): S70.

Kostis JB, Packer M, Black HR, et al. (2004). Omapatrilat and enalapril in patients with hypertension: the Omapatrilat Cardiovascular Treatment vs. Enalapril (OCTAVE) trial. *Am J Hypertens* **17**:103–11.

Llorens-Cortes C, Touyz R (2020). Evolution of a new class of antihypertensive drugs: targeting the brain renin–angiotensin system. *Hypertension* **75**:6–15.

Marc Y, Llorens-Cortes C (2011). The role of the brain renin–angiotensin system in hypertension: implications for new treatment. *Prog Neurobiol* **95**:89–103.

Wengenmayer C, Krikov M, Mueller S, et al. (2011). Novel therapy approach in primary stroke prevention: simultaneous inhibition of endothelin converting enzyme and neutral endopeptidase in spontaneously hypertensive, stroke-prone rats improves survival. *Neurol Res* **33**:201–7.

White WB, Weber MA, Sica D, et al. (2011). Effects of the angiotensin receptor blocker azilsartan medoxomil versus olmesartan and valsartan on ambulatory and clinic blood pressure in patients with stages 1 and 2 hypertension. *Hypertension* **57**:413–20.

CHAPTER 19

Renal denervation

Vikas Kapil

KEY POINTS

* Catheter-based renal denervation therapy offers an interventional approach to the control of blood pressure by aiming to disrupt both efferent and afferent sympathetic signalling between the cardiovascular control centres in the brainstem and the kidneys.
* Although initial trials were encouraging, a large sham-controlled study did not show any significant benefit.
* Newer techniques and catheters are currently being trialled and the results of these studies will determine whether or not this procedure will be part of management of hypertension in the years to come.

19.1 Introduction

Despite more than 60 years of therapeutic innovation and widespread access to low-cost, evidence-based pharmacological treatments for hypertension, raised blood pressure (BP) remains the leading modifiable risk factor for cardiovascular morbidity and mortality worldwide.

With the prevalence of hypertension expected to increase over time, novel strategies to lower BP in patients at risk of hypertension-related renal and vascular diseases are required. Whilst there is progress with the development of new classes of antihypertensive medications, one novel approach has been to target the autonomic nervous system through interventional techniques.

There is now a suite of technologies that have been successfully designed and are in clinical trials and/or clinical use, the most developed of which is renal (sympathetic) denervation. This chapter will outline the scientific basis for targeting autonomic neural signalling in the renal bed, and update with the latest clinical evidence regarding safety and efficacy. Lastly, the place for renal denervation in future guideline algorithms and further evidence required will be considered.

19.2 Rationale for renal denervation

The kidney is a highly innervated organ, with both efferent (from the brain to the kidney) and afferent (from the kidneys to the brain) sympathetic neurons innervating all essential kidney structures such as the juxtaglomerular apparatus and tubules, as well the renal vascular beds. Efferent sympathetic control of these kidney structures controls sodium and volume balance, as well as renin release, and are therefore key regulators of BP homeostasis. In addition to these crucial efferent sympathetically mediated effects, renal afferent nerves also signal to cardiovascular control centres in the central nervous system, thereby influencing efferent sympathetic neural control not only to the kidney itself, but also to other sympathetically innervated organs and structures involved in circulatory homeostasis.

The organotopic arrangement of sympathetic signalling (i.e. that neural traffic can be elevated relating to one organ system, but reduced or unchanged relating to others) has meant that establishing renal sympathetic signalling is increased in human hypertension and was no easy task to perform. However, the development of the regional radiolabelled noradrenaline spill-over technique by Professor Murray Esler's team from the Baker Institute, Melbourne provided clear evidence of enhanced renal sympathetic signalling and, with the above knowledge of the importance of both efferent and afferent signalling in BP regulation, made the renal nerves an attractive target for interventional technique development.

Whilst there is clear experimental evidence that renal denervation abrogates hypertension in various animal models of hypertension, even earlier approaches in malignant hypertension using surgical radical sympathectomy or splanchnicectomy resulted in impressive BP reduction and even reduction in mortality from this otherwise, at the time, rapidly fatal condition.

However, one cannot ascribe the benefit of such procedures to renal denervation alone, given the wide-ranging organ systems that were effectively denervated with such interventions and the procedures themselves had myriad problems, including procedural complications and post-operative orthostatic intolerance or hypotension. However, these studies, and later studies on patients with renal transplantation, reveal that denervated kidneys are able to handle sodium and water balance adequately and therefore provide a clear rationale for selective renal sympathectomy being both safe and efficacious.

19.3 Catheter-based renal denervation

To move the field forward required the development of a less-invasive, renal-selective technology that could interrupt renal neural signalling, whilst leaving other neural pathways intact and with minimal procedural complications. Taking advantage of the proposed proximity of the renal nerves to the adventitial surface of the renal arteries after they leave the paravertebral sympathetic chain, Ardian Inc. (now part of Medtronic) developed a catheter-based radiofrequency (RF) probe to heat the endothelial surface of the main renal artery to destroy the nerves running a few millimetres away on the adventitial side.

This first-generation RF ablation system was delivered retrogradely via the femoral artery access using a flexible (4-F) catheter to perform renal denervation with simultaneous rotation and withdrawal before each RF energy delivery; a helical pattern of endovascular treatments (4–6 per artery) was delivered to each artery.

The first-in-man observational study (SYMPLICITY HTN-1) in patients with resistant hypertension (where there was felt to be most need for additional therapies to lower BP) confirmed the safety and efficacy of this RF system, and was followed by the first multicentre, international randomized controlled study (SYMPLICITY HTN-2, $n = 106$). This study randomized patients with uncontrolled (office systolic BP >160 mmHg) resistant hypertension (>2 antihypertensive medications, including a diuretic) without concomitant moderate to severe chronic kidney disease (estimated glomerular filtration rate (eGFR) >45 mL/min/1.73 m^2) and with anatomically suitable renal arteries (no significant stenoses, >4 mm diameter, >20 mm main arterial length, single renal arteries) 1:1 to RF renal denervation plus medications or to medications alone. Mean difference between groups in changes in BP after 6 months were 32 mmHg and 8 mmHg for office and daytime ambulatory systolic BPs, respectively, favouring renal denervation.

These large effect sizes were unexpected and were responsible for a technological race to develop me-too solutions from different companies—at one point, over 30 catheter-based devices for renal denervation were in development or clinical testing. However, the neutral results of the first large placebo-controlled renal denervation study (SYMPLICITY HTN-3) caused a major contraction in the field, with most companies abandoning their clinical device development. SYMPLICITY HTN-3 was a US-based multicentre, randomized, placebo- (here preferred to the term 'sham', given the negative connotations outside of medicine with the word) controlled study, with similar inclusion criteria to SYMPLICITY HTN-2. Patients were randomized 2:1 to renal denervation or renal angiography alone, with attempts to mask the procedure to the patient to achieve blinding. Although there was a significant improvement from baseline in BP in the renal denervation group, this was matched by a surprising drop in BP in the placebo group.

Post hoc, there has been a great deal of effort from both technology companies and academics to explain the neutral result (i.e. the lack of between-group difference in change of BP) in SYMPLICITY HTN-3. Amazingly, only 6% of patients in the active renal denervation group had a procedure consistent with adequate circumferential ablation (i.e. enough RF burns to destroy the nerves in all directions around the artery) due to lack of adequate proctoring or technical experience with the procedure. Perhaps more tellingly, almost 40% of patients in both groups had changes in medications during the blinded follow-up phase, meaning that the magnitude of the real effect of renal denervation was still unknown. It is important to point out that this last criticism would apply to the earlier studies too.

19.4 New-generation catheters, techniques, and trials

The neutral result of SYMPLICITY HTN-3 and the methodological issues relating especially to unplanned changes in medications meant a period of reflection from academic triallists and technology companies alike. This period led to iteration and/or development of three advanced catheter systems currently in clinical trials, each employing unique properties: SPYRAL (Medtronic), PARADISE (ReCor Medical), and PEREGRINE (Ablative Solutions).

Whilst the SPYRAL catheter remains an RF catheter-based design, it has been refined to include multiple contact points along the length of the catheter, which curls up once deployed in the renal artery and allows a single energy delivery period to simultaneously ablate in discrete sections of the renal artery to provide a 360° ablation field.

The PARADISE catheter is an intravascular catheter containing a low-pressure, water-filled cooling balloon comprising an ultrasound emitter which emits ultrasonic energy in a 360° pattern to heat distant tissue at a distance of 1–6 mm, achieving a contiguous circumferential ring of ablation damage.

The PEREGRINE catheter takes a different approach to using energy (either RF or ultrasound) by deploying three microneedles once in the renal artery lumen. These microneedles pierce the renal arterial wall and allow injection of concentrated ethanol as a neurolytic on the outside of the renal artery where the renal nerves run to/from the kidney.

Just as importantly as advancements in catheter technology was a reappraisal of the human renal nerve anatomy, which one should argue should have come before the deployment of first-in-man technologies. Whilst the original concept was that the renal nerves are closest to the adventitial arterial wall proximally as they leave the sympathetic chain/ganglia and begin to diverge away from the arterial wall towards the renal pole, meaning that first-generation catheters and trials were designed to be deployed in the proximal main renal artery, more recent histopathological studies have confirmed the opposite—the renal nerves are at closest apposition to the renal arteries close to the renal hilum at the renal arterial branches. If the renal nerves are targeted distally, by using catheters that can be manipulated into the main bifurcations of the renal arteries, then renal denervation is more efficacious, at least when axonal damage and renal noradrenaline content are the markers of success in swine.

Following these technical advancements, there remained a clear mandate to answer one clinical question: what is the true effect of renal denervation on BP?

The way to answer this in the clearest, most unambiguous way is in a placebo-controlled, blinded, randomized study of hypertensive patients on *no* medications, thereby removing the issues of possible medication changes. Use of ambulatory BP as the primary entry criterion and primary endpoint helps with numerous bias issues with using office BP and helps reduce uncertainty over effect size by using numerous readings (at least 14 during daytime) for the endpoint in each person. However, the fact that patients have uncontrolled, unmedicated hypertension means that these trials were done in a lower-risk population than the earlier trials (level of uncontrolled BP not as severe as in patients in SYMPLICITY HTN 1–3, for example) and the follow-up period was considerably shorter for the blinded analysis period (2–3 months of being on no medication post-randomization and intervention/placebo intervention). The off-medication studies are similar for both the SPYRAL and PARADISE programmes—patients either off medications at baseline or washed out of up to two antihypertensives, with further urine assessments of compliance to staying off medications for the duration of follow-up in the blinded assessment period.

In conjunction with off-medication studies, more clinically meaningful studies alongside this are needed in patients who fail to achieve BP control despite guideline-based pharmacotherapy. Therefore, protocol-driven on-medication studies of patients with 6-month primary endpoint follow-up have been designed with a urine-based assay of medication adherence used to determine medication stability. The SPYRAL ON MED pilot trial used a hypertension population on 1–3 medications, all at least on 50% of the recommended dose (half of patients on three medications), whilst A Study of the ReCor Medical Paradise System in Clinical Hypertension (RADIANCE TRIO) (using the PARADISE catheter) used a fixed-dose triple-combination medication containing guideline-based therapy (thiazide diuretic, calcium channel blocker, and angiotensin receptor blocker).

Whilst the off-medication studies have been reported in final form, the on-medication studies have been slower to recruit and RADIANCE TRIO has only been press-released as of writing, with no pre-print or peer-reviewed abstract or manuscript to read, and the SPYRAL ON MED programme has only completed the proof-of-concept pilot study, with the SPYRAL ON MED EXPANSION study still ongoing, which will use Bayesian priors from the pilot study in the final analysis, as was done with the SPYRAL OFF MED -PIVOTAL studies.

From the off-medication studies, it is clear that the magnitude of effect from early open-label or non-placebo-controlled renal denervation studies was exaggerated by various biases; the real placebo-corrected magnitude of effect of renal denervation in patients with stage I/II hypertension (baseline 24-hour ambulatory BP: 143/88 mmHg for RADIANCE SOLO; and 151/98 mmHg for SPYRAL OFF MED PIVOTAL) is closer to 5 mmHg ambulatory systolic BP, rather than 30 mmHg, as per SYMPLICITY HTN-1 and HTN-2 (Figure 19.1, top panels). Furthermore, from the only data we have seen to date from the on-medication studies, the magnitude of effect in patient on medications is similar at around approximately 7 mmHg (Figure 19.1 bottom panel). In most studies, 5–7 mmHg of 24-hour ambulatory systolic BP reduction would equate to approximately 10 mmHg of office systolic BP reduction, which is similar in magnitude to the effect of a single antihypertensive medication in mild hypertension.

19.5 Issues to be resolved

Whilst the recent trials have given some much-needed clarity as to the magnitude of effect of renal denervation being approximate to that of a single medication, other important questions are yet to be fully answered.

19.5.1 Durability of BP lowering

The newly designed and published trials described above have shown BP lowering in patients on no medications up to 2–3 months post-renal

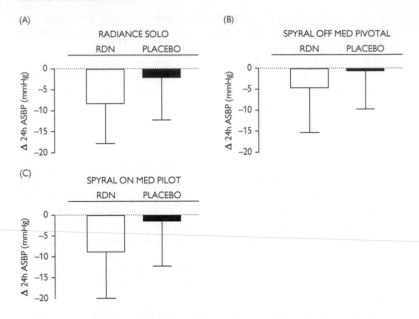

Figure 19.1 Change in 24-hour ambulatory systolic blood pressure from baseline in recent second-generation renal denervation studies. Top panel (A) and (B) shows off-medication studies with the primary endpoint measured at 2 or 3 months, respectively. Panel (C) shows on-medication study with the primary endpoint measured at 6 months.

Δ, change from baseline; 24h, 24 hour; ASBP, ambulatory systolic blood pressure; RDN, renal denervation.

denervation and up to 6 months in patients on medications. Due to the inherent cardiovascular risk of leaving patients untreated or undertreated, it is not ethical to keep patients off more medications for longer, therefore not allowing long-term evaluation of the effect of renal denervation that is not complicated by medication effects. The longest-term data from the Global SYMPLICITY registry in >300 patients followed up for 3 years with repeated ambulatory BP measurements show no diminution of effect over time, with mean ambulatory SBP reduction of approximately 8 mmHg, similar to the placebo-controlled off- and on-medication studies described earlier, though in the registry study, there is clearly an inability to control for medication changes over time as well.

19.5.2 Who should receive renal denervation?

Given the heterogenous response to renal denervation, as can be seen by the standard deviations in Figure 19.1, there have been some suggestions that we should select patients in clinical practice for renal denervation who are most likely to have a large response, given that techniques to establish elevated renal sympathetic signalling are far from mainstream clinical tests. From the data collected so far, the only reliable indicators of a large response appear to be a higher baseline BP (as is common also to all antihypertensive medications) and combined hypertension (i.e. systolo-diastolic hypertension, in contrast to isolated systolic hypertension), perhaps reflecting that in situations of advanced arterial stiffness (largely the cause of isolated systolic hypertension), elevated sympathetic signalling is not a predominant driver to hypertension.

In most health economies, renal denervation is not well established, in line with the UK Joint Societies' recommendation of continuing the moratorium on renal denervation as routine clinical care, pending further evidence. Whether trials with hard endpoints, similar to seminal antihypertensive medication studies, to demonstrate a reduction in cardiovascular morbidity and mortality are required is not clear from European or North American regulatory agencies and the conduct of such a trial would be very difficult to pursue, given the ethical need to treat to target, given the well-established evidence base for antihypertensive therapy and BP thresholds. However, it may be possible to design a non-inferiority trial with randomization to renal denervation as part of a strategy to get to controlled BP. If the groups with similar achieved BP have similar morbidity and mortality over time, then we could ascribe the same beneficial effect from BP lowering from renal denervation to that of medications (assuming there was a difference between groups in medication burden).

Furthermore, whether there is a place for patient choice (choosing a procedure over an extra medication) is a further dilemma for health economies to decide, but it is important to reiterate that for most patients, renal denervation would not control stage I/II hypertension on its own, given the observed magnitude of effect, and therefore could be considered a very expensive, "long acting" antihypertensive medications, with effects lasting at least 3 years. Given that most guideline-based medications for hypertension are available in generic formulation, the health economics of this approach are not favourable.

19.5.3 Safety of renal denervation

One of the big concerns regarding renal denervation has been both procedural and long-term renal safety. Whilst in the most recent trials, there were no procedural safety events, they however, reported a low incidence of vascular access site injury occurring at a rate of 1–2%. Although there have been sporadic reports of renal artery stenosis occurring post-renal denervation, this has not been observed routinely during active surveillance up to 6 months post-procedure more recently with second-generation catheters. Furthermore, there is no evidence of a deleterious effect on renal function, either with protocol-driven follow-up or in longer-term (>3 years) registry follow-up.

19.6 Conclusion

Renal denervation has been established as an interventional approach to improve BP control. It seems to have a device agnostic effect similar to a single BP medication, with durable and safe results up to 3 years post-procedure. How health economies integrate this new treatment into existing treatment algorithms, alongside cheap, generic medications, is yet to be established.

KEY REFERENCES

Azizi M, Schmieder RE, Mahfoud F, et al. (2018). Endovascular ultrasound renal denervation to treat hypertension (RADIANCE-HTN SOLO): a multicentre, international, single-blind, randomised, sham-controlled trial. Lancet 391:2335–45.

Bhatt DL, Kandzari DE, O'Neill WW, et al. (2014). A controlled trial of renal denervation for resistant hypertension. N Engl J Med 370:1393–401.

Böhm M, Kario K, Kandzari DE, et al. (2020). Efficacy of catheter-based renal denervation in the absence of antihypertensive medications (SPYRAL HTN-OFF MED Pivotal): a multicentre, randomised, sham-controlled trial. Lancet 395:1444–51.

DiBona GF (2004). The sympathetic nervous system and hypertension: recent developments. Hypertension 43:147–50.

Esler MD, Krum H, Sobotka PA, et al. (2010). Renal sympathetic denervation in patients with treatment-resistant hypertension (the Symplicity HTN-2 trial): a randomised controlled trial. Lancet 376:1903–9.

GBD 2017 Risk Factor Collaborators (2018). Global, regional, and national comparative risk assessment of 84 behavioural, environmental and occupational, and metabolic risks or clusters of risks for 195 countries and territories, 1990–2017: a systematic analysis for the Global Burden of Disease Study 2017. Lancet 392:1923–94.

Kandzari DE, Bohm M, Mahfoud F, et al. (2018). Effect of renal denervation on blood pressure in the presence of antihypertensive drugs: 6-month efficacy and safety results from the SPYRAL HTN-ON MED proof-of-concept randomised trial. Lancet 391:2346–55.

Lobo MD, Sobotka PA, Pathak A, et al. (2016). Interventional procedures and future drug therapy for hypertension. Eur Heart J 38:1101–11.

Lobo MD, Sharp ASP, Kapil V, et al. (2019). Joint UK societies' 2019 consensus statement on renal denervation. Heart 105:1456–63.

Mahfoud F, Bohm M, Schmieder R, et al. (2019). Effects of renal denervation on kidney function and long-term outcomes: 3-year follow-up from the Global SYMPLICITY Registry. Eur Heart J 40:3474–82.

Sharp AS, Davies JE, Lobo MD, et al. (2016). Renal artery sympathetic denervation: observations from the UK experience. Clin Res Cardiol 105:544–52.

Improving medication adherence in hypertension

Hassan Al-Riyami and Deirdre A. Lane

KEY POINTS

* Adherence to medications and prescribed non-pharmacological interventions is key to optimal blood pressure control in patients with hypertension and is associated with better cardiovascular outcomes.

* Patients should be questioned regarding adherence to therapy at each visit, especially if blood pressure appears to be uncontrolled.

* Many factors contribute to non-adherence (patient- and healthcare system-related), and an understanding of factors pertinent to the individual patient is key to improving their adherence.

* Improving adherence requires a multidisciplinary approach with use of community healthcare workers, nurses, and pharmacists and involvement of patients and their caregivers in all decisions undertaken.

20.1 Introduction

For patients with hypertension, adherence to antihypertensive medications and lifestyle changes is key to controlling their blood pressure (BP). However, as with other chronic illnesses, non-adherence to medication remains a major issue. Although recent data appear to suggest that in some countries, such as the United States and Canada, rates of BP control are improving (thereby suggesting better adherence to medications), data from most other countries reveal persistently high numbers of patients with uncontrolled BP, reflecting poor adherence to medication and recommended lifestyle modifications.

The reported rates of adherence to antihypertensive medications vary from as low as 32% to around 68%. There are data to suggest that at the end of 6 months, one-third of patients discontinue their antihypertensive medications and only around half of all patients persist with their initial therapy at 1 year. Studies have also shown that a sizeable proportion of patients labelled as having 're-sistant hypertension' or 'poorly controlled/uncontrolled hypertension' are ac-tually non-adherent to medications. Uncontrolled or poorly controlled BP is a major health concern as it is associated with higher cardiovascular mortality and morbidity. Indeed, the World Health Organization (WHO), in its report on ad-herence to long-term therapies, states that interventions to improve medication adherence might have a far greater impact on the health of the population than any improvement in a specific medical treatment itself. Medication adherence is associated with improved cost savings and helps advancements in medical technology achieve their full potential and ultimately reduces the burden of chronic illnesses. Early detection of non-adherence can prevent expensive investigations and unnecessary additional medications and interventions. Ensuring medication adherence is essential, given that the latest hypertension guidelines have lowered the BP treatment targets, and achieving these targets requires good medication adherence.

There have been many definitions of medical adherence, but the WHO definition is the most widely used. It is defined as the extent to which a person's behaviour (i.e. taking medication, following a diet, and executing lifestyle changes) corresponds to agreed recommendations from a healthcare provider. Adherence is an independent, active, voluntary, and collaborative involvement of the patient, resulting in them taking a range of actions to produce a desired therapeutic result that has been agreed upon by the patient and the healthcare provider. Although erroneously used interchangeably, adherence differs from 'compliance' as the latter implies that the patient passively accepts the recommendations of the prescriber, with little or no engagement by the patient themselves.

According to the Ascertaining Barriers to Compliance (ABC) project team, adherence to medications involves acceptance and execution of the decisions made by the prescriber. It includes *initiation* of the treatment, *implementation* of the prescribed regime, and *discontinuation* of the pharmacotherapy when recommended. The term 'primary non-adherence' has been used to refer to cases where the patient fails to initiate therapy either as a result of non-acceptance of the diagnosis (denial) or due to fear of side effects or other personal reasons. Conversely, secondary non-adherence refers to patients who have accepted the diagnosis and commenced medications, but then become irregular users or even permanently stop taking their medications midway through the course of their therapy. Non-adherence can also be classified as purposeful or non-intentional, based on whether the patient is intentionally not taking their prescribed medications or whether it results from forgetfulness or cognitive impairment.

20.2 Factors affecting adherence

The degree of adherence to medication by any individual patient can change over time and is dependent on many factors. Unlike most other conditions, patients with hypertension are often asymptomatic. Here, the absence of symptoms and the fear of side effects from medications contribute significantly to non-adherence to antihypertensives. Many patients argue that they have no symptoms yet must take medications daily that can then cause symptoms and adverse side effects.

The WHO has identified five broad categories of factors that affect adherence: (1) socio-economic factors; (2) patient-related; (3) therapy-related; (4) comorbid conditions; and (5) healthcare system-related (Figure 20.1). These factors are

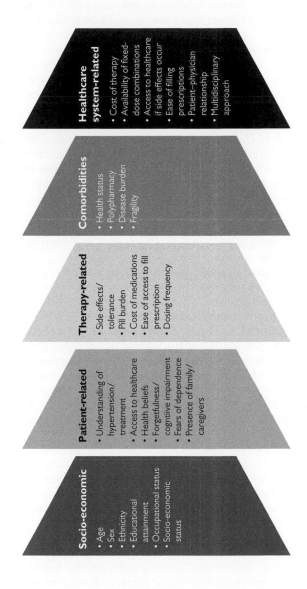

Figure 20.1 Factors affecting medication adherence.

Socio-economic
- Age
- Sex
- Ethnicity
- Educational attainment
- Occupational status
- Socio-economic status

Patient-related
- Understanding of hypertension/treatment
- Access to healthcare
- Health beliefs
- Forgetfulness/cognitive impairment
- Fears of dependence
- Presence of family/caregivers

Therapy-related
- Side effects/tolerance
- Pill burden
- Cost of medications
- Ease of access to fill prescription
- Dosing frequency

Comorbidities
- Health status
- Polypharmacy
- Disease burden
- Fragility

Healthcare system-related
- Cost of therapy
- Availability of fixed-dose combinations
- Access to healthcare if side effects occur
- Ease of filling prescriptions
- Patient–physician relationship
- Multidisciplinary approach

interdependent and ultimately play a role in the individual patient's willingness or ability to be adherent to medications. Socio-economic factors, such as age, sex, ethnicity, social, economic, educational, and occupational status, can affect adherence in many ways. These have a bearing on patient-related factors such as their understanding of the disease, access to healthcare, health beliefs, forgetfulness, and fears of dependence. Therapy-related factors and comorbid conditions reflect the total pill burden on the patient, side effects, cost of medications, and the ease of access to medications and refills. This is also related to the healthcare system factors which determine the cost of therapy, the availability of fixed-dose combinations, access to healthcare in case of side effects, and the ease of filling prescriptions, etc.

Patients' beliefs and fears regarding the diagnosis and impact of this diagnosis on their lifestyle also play a role in adherence. In some countries, the diagnosis of a chronic illness, such as hypertension, may have an impact on their health insurance and job prospects, leading to some patients denying that anything is wrong with them, and therefore not taking their medications. In some cultures, there is a suspicion towards modern medicine, with a tendency to try traditional therapies first. Side effects, such as postural hypotension in the elderly, erectile dysfunction, and frequent micturition, may also limit acceptance of, and adherence to, medication by some patients.

Several psychological theories have been postulated which relate to health beliefs and behaviours, ultimately determining adherence/non-adherence. The 'health beliefs model' proposes that patients weigh up the costs/benefits of a health-related behaviour (be it lifestyle changes or adherence to medications), based on their perceived susceptibility to the disease, its seriousness, and the potential benefits and costs (e.g. side effects, financial, etc.) of changing and sustaining the new health-promoting behaviour. Other factors, such as current health status, demographic factors (age, sex, ethnicity, cultural factors), and external influences such as family/caregivers and healthcare providers, also contribute to the likelihood of behavioural change and adherence. An alternate theory is the theory of planned behaviour, which describes action as secondary to intention, with intention derived from personal attitudes and influenced by the views of significant others (e.g. family/caregivers, general practitioners/family doctors, etc.). The self-regulatory model proposes that health-related behaviours are strongly influenced by ideas about the illness and these beliefs determine an individual's coping strategies, including adherence to medications, assess the likely success of their treatment, and determine whether it will be beneficial to continue treatment or not.

20.3 Assessment of adherence

Due to its effects on the individual patient and the potential burden of uncontrolled BP on the healthcare system as a whole, assessment of adherence to medications in all hypertensive patients is extremely important, especially when the prescribed drug therapy appears to be ineffective and where the physician is inclined to increase or change the drug regimen. Non-adherence to medications should be ruled out in patients who are labelled as having 'resistant hypertension' before specialist referral. In clinical practice, however, assessment of suboptimal medication adherence is challenging, due to the dynamic nature of adherence where the patient will have periods of varying levels of adherence/non-adherence, depending on their personal situation. In addition, there is no clear gold standard method of assessing adherence. Similarly, there is no set criterion to determine what level of adherence is considered as 'good adherence' or 'bad adherence'.

The most common method of assessing medication adherence used in daily clinical practice is direct patient questioning based on self-recall and self-reporting. This method is, however, very unreliable and multiple studies have shown that patients and physicians tend to overreport medication adherence, with some authors stating that this method is no better than the toss of a coin.

Use of standard structured questionnaires is another method often utilized in clinical trials and has been recommended to be used in daily clinical practice. However, lack of time and the nature of these questions often limit the practicality of their use at each clinic visit. There are many questionnaires available and some such as the Hill–Bone Compliance Scale are specifically tailored for use in hypertensive patients. Table 20.1 summarizes some of these widely available questionnaires, along with their advantages and disadvantages. The updated eight-item Morisky Medication Adherence Scale (MMAS-8) and the Self-efficacy for Appropriate Medication Use (SEAMS) questionnaire have high internal consistency and are frequently used. These questionnaires are good as screening tools as they provide a sense of the level of adherence, but they do not delve into the causes behind non-adherence.

Other indirect methods include pill count where patients bring their medications to consultations and the physician or health care professionals (HCP) counts the number of tablets remaining. This is the method used often in clinical trials, but it is time-consuming, and therefore often not practical in daily clinical practice and infrequently implemented. Measuring the number of refill prescriptions issued to patients works in a similar manner where patients who are strictly adherent to medications will often get a refill prescription ahead of when the previous one expires. Use of electronic health records and pharmacy databases can help to highlight patients who have missed appointments or have not collected their refill prescriptions on time.

The directly observed method was popularized in many countries for treatment of diseases of public health interest such as tuberculosis and leprosy. Here health workers would administer the medications directly under their supervision and maintain strict pill counts. Under these conditions, treatment is for a relatively short duration and therefore may not be practical for chronic illnesses such as hypertension. It could, however, be tried in a small subset of patients with resistant hypertension and very high BP where non-adherence might be suspected. In these cases, the patient could be admitted to supervise medication intake.

CHAPTER 20

Table 20.1 Commonly used questionnaires to assess adherence to treatment in patients with chronic illnesses

Questionnaire	Features/advantages	Disadvantages	Validated conditions for use
MMAS-8 (Morisky et al., 2008)	• Eight questions • High internal consistency (Cronbach's alpha 0.83) • High sensitivity and specificity (93% and 53%, respectively) • Available in many languages (e.g. French, Portuguese, Urdu, Turkish, Chinese, Malay) • Useful as a screening tool • Easy to use; quick (approximately 1 minute)	• Does not fully explore factors contributing to non-adherence	• Hypertension • Hyperlipidaemia • Diabetes mellitus • Parkinson's disease • Heart failure • Ischaemic heart disease
HBCS (Hill et al., 1995)	• 14 questions • High internal consistency (Cronbach's alpha 0.79) • Sensitivity and specificity of 67.4% and 67.8%, respectively • Available in many languages (e.g. Arabic, Chinese, German, Korean, Malay, Persian, Polish, Portuguese, Turkish) • Identifies barriers to adherence • Includes questions related to salt intake	• Developed specifically for hypertension and African ethnicity • Validated in other conditions, although questions are fairly hypertension-specific • Not validated in other ethnicities • Time-consuming (approximately 5 minutes, compared to other questionnaires)	• Hypertension • Diabetes mellitus • Stroke • Human immunodeficiency virus
SEAMS (Riser et al., 2007)	• 13 questions • High internal consistency (Cronbach's alpha 0.89) • Based on the socio-cognitive theory • Can be used in patients with limited literacy • Identifies barriers to adherence	• Time-consuming (approximately 5 minutes) • Not practical for everyday use	• Ischaemic heart disease • Hypertension • Diabetes mellitus
BMQ (Svarstad et al., 1999)	• 2- to 5-item scales • Short and easy to use (approximately 1 minute) • Available in many languages (e.g. Swedish, Malay, Dutch, Spanish, Maltese) • Sensitivity and specificity of 77% and 58%, respectively • Assesses patients' beliefs and attitudes towards their condition specifically and medications in general	• Does not identify barriers to non-adherence • Low internal consistency, compared to the other questionnaires (Cronbach's alpha 0.66)	• Diabetes mellitus • Hypertension

BMQ, Beliefs about Medicines Questionnaire; HBCS, Hill–Bone Compliance Scale; MMAS, Morisky Medication Adherence Scale; SEAMS, Self-efficacy for Appropriate Medication Use.

Measuring the level of drugs or their metabolites in the plasma or urine is often used in drug trials. However, in daily clinical practice, these are cumbersome and expensive, and therefore not always practical. Urinalysis of most commonly used antihypertensives is available and their complete absence in a spot urine sample can suggest total non-adherence.

Some new technology such as electronic monitoring systems are being trialled. Here microcircuits embedded in medication packaging keep a record of the number of doses that are taken, along with the date and time. This would accurately record when the tablet is removed from the packaging but is open to manipulation by the patient (i.e. removed from the package, but not consumed). The Proteus device™ (Proteus Digital Health, Redwood City, CA, USA) is an innovative method that incorporates an ingestible sensor, along with the tablet itself. The ingested sensor is activated in the stomach and the signal is picked up by a skin patch, which is then transmitted to a bluetooth-enabled device. Results of the trials are promising and this might be the future of adherence monitoring. At present, however, these emerging technologies are expensive and not readily available. Once commercially available, they might initially have a limited role in patients with resistant hypertension where non-adherence is suspected.

20.4 Strategies to improve adherence

During the brief clinical encounter in a busy outpatient setting, it is difficult to get a true sense of the level of adherence to medication and the factors that might prevent a patient from being fully adherent to prescribed medications. However, the physician should be vigilant in picking up clues pointing to non-adherence such as missed appointments, late prescription refill, higher-than-usual blood pressure, etc.

Adherence is a very individual characteristic and often members of the same household will exhibit different levels of adherence. It may also vary in the same patient at different times. Therefore, ascertaining the reasons for non-adherence in each patient and assessing their beliefs and concerns regarding their diagnosis and management play an important part in improving adherence. Healthcare professionals can help patients overcome many of the barriers to adherence by working in collaboration with their patients and family members/caregivers and other providers to identify, remove, or minimize the barriers. Discussions with the patient and their caregiver should be open, with a non-confrontational 'no-blame' approach, to come to a common agreed plan.

Whilst there is no single gold standard strategy for improving adherence, it is generally recognized that using multi-pronged individualized interventions is the best approach. The strategies used to improve adherence will depend on the five categories of factors that affect adherence mentioned earlier (Figure 20.2). First and foremost, it is important to understand and try to view things from the perspective of the patient. For most patients, forgetfulness plays a major part in non-adherence. Those with busy lifestyles might find it difficult to remember

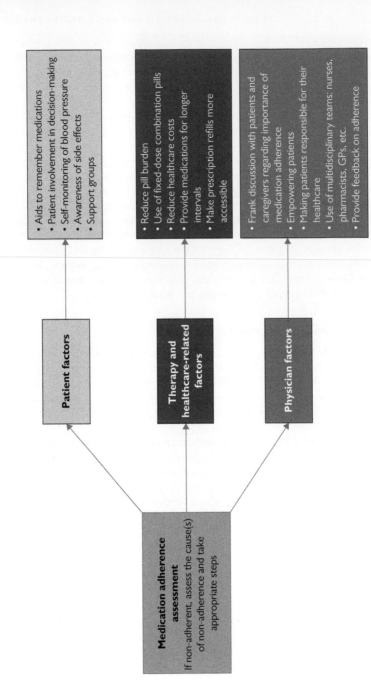

Figure 20.2 Strategies to improve patient medication adherence.

and it is important to educate the patient on the need for, and importance of, adherence. Side effects should be explained in detail, so the patient will know what to expect and how some side effects could be ameliorated. Aids to remind the patient to take their medications, such as daily text messages, email alerts or entries in the diary, dosette-boxes, etc., depending on patient preferences, can help. Associating medication intake with a particular daily activity, for example, to take it with breakfast, can help the patient remember. In patients with cognitive impairment, the responsibility for administering medication could be transferred to their caregiver, who ought to be educated on the importance of medication adherence and the regimen required.

Involvement of a multidisciplinary team that includes pharmacists, specialist nurses, community healthcare workers, general practitioners/family doctors, and hypertension specialists can have a positive impact on increasing medication adherence. During each visit or contact with the patient, adherence to medication should be discussed. The team-based care approach allows patients to feel they have more than one healthcare professional to whom they can turn in case of any problems with their medications. In addition, pharmacists and nurses have been shown to be more effective in providing high-quality patient education than hospital-based physicians who are often more time-constrained. Involvement of the patient and family/caregivers in decision-making, in terms of choice of drug (and their potential side effects such as increased diuresis with diuretics), timing of medications, etc., helps to improve adherence. Similarly, involving the patient in home monitoring of BP has been shown to be effective in improving adherence. Home monitoring provides the patient with immediate feedback regarding their BP and also serves as a reminder to be adherent to medications. Empowering the patient to take more responsibility for their BP control and management by self-monitoring can also improve medication adherence.

Use of fixed-dose combination pills that lower the number of tablets that need to be consumed would be helpful for patients with multiple comorbidities who have a high daily pill burden. Studies have shown that non-adherence is around 10% with one pill daily and 20% with two pills daily, resulting in very high rates (>40%) of partial or complete non-adherence in patients receiving five or more pills daily. Use of cheaper generic medications may also be useful if cost is a contributing factor to non-adherence. Synchronizing medication refills, along with providing longer supplies, can help those with busy schedules. Other approaches for improving adherence that have been implemented with some success include cognitive behavioural therapy and motivational interviewing.

Modern technology can also play a role in improving adherence to medication. Use of electronic applications on smart phones or devices to remind patients to take their medications has been demonstrated to be effective in many clinical settings. Use of electronic medication packaging devices that monitor adherence can also serve as a reminder to improve adherence; being aware that they are being monitored might encourage patients to be more adherent. Some patients may find that being part of a social network and self-help groups is beneficial in helping to improve adherence.

20.5 Conclusion

Adherence to medications is an integral part of management of hypertension. Better communication between the healthcare provider and the patient and their caregiver is key to understanding the barriers to medication adherence and overcoming these obstacles. The treating physician should be sensitive to the individual needs of the patient, so that therapy can be tailored according to their personal circumstances. Improving adherence requires a multi-pronged approach with multidisciplinary team involvement and complete engagement of the patient or their caregiver. As has been demonstrated in some countries, high levels of adherence is possible with investment in time and effort by the physician, which will result in significant health benefits for the patient and the population as a whole.

KEY REFERENCES

Burnier M, Egan BM (2019). Adherence in hypertension: a review of prevalence, risk factors, impact and management. *Circ Res* **124**:1124–40.

Chang TE, Ritchey MD, Ayala C, Durthaler JM, Loustalot F (2018). Use of strategies to improve antihypertensive medication adherence within United States outpatient health care practices, DocStyles 2015–2016. *J Clin Hypertens* **20**:225–32.

Hafezi H, Robertson TL, Moon DG, Au-Yeung K, Zdeblick MJ, Savage GM (2015). An ingestible sensor for measuring medication adherence. *IEEE Trans Biomed Eng* **62**:99–109.

Kubica A, Kosobucka A, Michalskil P, Fabiszak T, Felsmann M (2017). Self-reported questionnaires for assessment adherence to treatment in patients with cardiovascular diseases. *Med Res J* **2**:115–22.

The ABC Project Team (2012). Ascertaining barriers for compliance: policies for safe, effective and cost-effective use of medicines in Europe. Final report of the ABC Project 2012. Available from: http://abcproject.eu/img/ABC%20Final.pdf

Vrijens B, De Geest S, Hughes DA, *et al*.; ABC Project Team (2012). A new taxonomy for describing and defining adherence to medications. *Br J Clin Pharmacol* **73**:691–705.

World Health Organization (2003). Adherence to long term therapies: evidence for action. Geneva: World Health Organization. Available from: http://apps.who.int/iris/bitstream/handle/10665/42682/9241545992.pdf;jsessionid=1949C18B4AC24293F FAC7B05D002C338?sequence=1

Part 4
Special conditions

Hypertension in pregnancy: physiopathological, preventive, therapeutic, and long-term considerations

Gloria Valdés

KEY POINTS

- Evaluation, management, and follow-up of hypertensive pregnancies must always contemplate the benefit of the mother and her offspring.
- Pre-eclampsia is a syndrome, not a disease, as it derives from a combination of different physiopathological pathways.
- In pre-eclamptic patients, antihypertensive treatment protects the mother from acute target organ damage but does not modify the course of a multifactorial condition.
- A hypertensive pregnancy should be considered a positive stress test that represents a window of opportunity to initiate early cardiovascular prevention.
- An unfavourable uterine environment increases the risk of future cardiovascular, metabolic, and renal diseases that therefore require long-term follow-up.

21.1 Introduction

Hypertensive disorders of pregnancy (HDP) affect approximately 10% of gestations and represent the most frequent medical complication of pregnancy and early post-partum period, and present with diverse causes and clinical expressions. Understanding their pathophysiology, prevention, clinical expression, and therapeutic management enables early detection in order to reduce maternal and fetal complications (Table 21.1) and to prolong pregnancy with minimum risk to the mother and her offspring. In addition, their long-term evolution should prompt surveillance of cardiovascular risks in the mother and deficits in intrauterine programming in the child.

21.2 Classification

Classification, as well as many of the recommendations in this chapter, derives from the 2018 guidelines of the International Society for the Study of

Table 21.1 Maternal, fetal, and neonatal risks of hypertensive disorders of pregnancy

Maternal	Fetal and neonatal
Placental abruption	Preterm birth
Cardiac and renal failure	Intrauterine growth restriction
Subendocardial necrosis	Fetal vasocontriction
Liver dysfunction	Heart failure
Disseminated intravascular coagulation	Subendocardial necrosis
Stroke	Fetal or neonatal death
Eclampsia	
Death	

Hypertension in Pregnancy (ISSHP), a living document planned to incorporate findings with clinical impact on a field that constitutes work in progress.

1. Pre-eclampsia–eclampsia is a syndrome, not a disease, since its aetiologies and manifestations are multifactorial. It represents a great risk for mother and child, which increases with recurrent pre-eclampsia (PE) or presents in multiparas. PE is conventionally defined as de novo hypertension and proteinuria beyond the 20th gestational week. The diagnosis of PE in the absence of proteinuria has been currently widened to include neurological, hepatic, haematological, renal, and fetal damage. Because of its unpredictable evolution, the classification of mild and severe PE has been replaced by PE and PE with severe features. Another subdivision is determined by early or late onset, according to a cut-off point at the 34th gestational week; the former being associated with PE with severe features.

The HELLP syndrome (haemolysis, elevated liver enzymes, low platelets) has either a sudden onset or may start with severe thrombocytopenia and hepatic dysfunction that, in a second phase, presents with hypertension and proteinuria. Eclampsia is the most intense form, as endothelial dysfunction, blood pressure increment, and vasoconstriction cause encephalopathy derived from oedema, haemorrhages, and infarctions, resulting in convulsions. Eclampsia reappears in 1–2% and around 22–35% of patients present with recurrent PE.

2. Chronic essential or secondary hypertension accounts for approximately 25% of pregnant hypertensive women, and is characterized by its pre-gestational diagnosis, or if blood pressure was not measured previously, it may emerge during gestation. It can cause intrauterine growth restriction.

3. Chronic essential or secondary hypertension with superimposed PE presents with a 5-fold risk, compared to normal women. Maternal and fetal risks are increased by the magnitude of the underlying hypertension, glomerular filtration rate of <40 mL/min, secondary renal hypertension, or proteinuria of >1 g/day. After gestational week 20, blood pressure increases, proteinuria appears or previous values rise, hyperuricaemia is observed, and thrombocytopenia and increased hepatic enzymes predate the HELLP syndrome.

4. Gestational hypertension is a non-proteinuric blood pressure elevation that recurs in subsequent pregnancies at earlier gestational stages. In the median and long term, 40–60% of cases develop essential hypertension.

5. Transient hypertension defines a blood pressure rise that disappears in sequential determinations along the same visit. The risk of gestational hypertension or PE is 40%.

6. White coat hypertension represents the reactivity of the patient. It is confirmed by ambulatory blood pressure monitoring or home blood pressures.

7. Masked hypertension may be due to lower office values than in ordinary life or to previous hypertension that disappears due to the vasodilator surge of early pregnancy. It is suspected from normal pressures with target organ damage and is confirmed similarly to white coat hypertension.

In the majority of cases, the clinical history and a basic laboratory workup will permit the differential diagnosis; in a few cases, post-partum evolution will define a diagnostic certainty. When in doubt, it is better to suspect isolated or superimposed PE, due to its uncertain evolution and the fetal risk derived from a fragile placenta.

21.3 Physiological and pathological gestational adaptation

21.3.1 Normal pregnancy

To better understand the physiopathology and appropriate management of PE–eclampsia and other HDP, it is necessary to recognize the changes of haemodynamic and vasoactive factors in normal pregnancy. In the first place, the pregnant woman retains 500 mEq of sodium and 4–5 L of water due to increased aldosterone levels and vascular compliance; these expand the plasma volume, which is accompanied by a physiological decrease in the haematocrit. Cardiac output increases progressively and surpasses by 30–40% the normal levels at 24–28 gestational weeks. Plasma renin activity and angiotensinogen levels are elevated, but reactivity to exogenous angiotensin II is reduced. In spite of variations in factors that increase blood pressure, this paradoxically remains normal or slightly decreases due to a reduction in peripheral resistance provoked by a surge of vasodilator factors. If available, the difference between pre-gestational and early pregnancy blood pressures helps predict maternal cardiovascular adaptability. Among the vasodilators, nitric oxide occupies a central role, in interaction with prostacyclin, prostaglandin E2, angiotensin (1-7), bradykinin, and vascular endothelial growth factor (VEGF). In the utero-placental interface, this vasodilator network contributes to extravillous trophoblast (EVT) invasion and placental angiogenesis. Up to week 22, the EVT replaces the smooth muscle of the spiral arteries and transforms them into non-reactive saccular conduits that permit blood to enter the intervillous space at low velocity. Maternal and fetal blood are separated by a barrier that becomes thinner as pregnancy and fetal requirements increase; this is constituted by the endothelium of the villous capillaries, the villous stroma, and the syncytiotrophoblast. The syncytiotrophoblast—a single cell that constitutes the 'placental endothelium'—is under constant regeneration and sheds 2–3 g of apoptotic material per day into maternal circulation, provoking low-grade inflammation.

21.3.2 Pre-eclampsia–eclampsia

21.3.2.1 Initial silent stage

In the early 1970s, Brosens, Robertson, and Dixon observed a deficient invasion of the spiral arteries by the EVT. Currently, several pathways affect arterial remodelling (inherent to decidualization, the trophoblast, immunological tolerance, decreased arterial receptivity due to endothelial dysfunction, and arteriolosclerosis). Apart from increased pulsatility of the uterine arteries detected by ultrasound, this phase is clinically silent.

21.3.2.2 Systemic phase

The role of apoptotic particles, exosomes, microvesicles, cell-free fetal DNA, and soluble factors derived from the syncytiotrophoblast shedd into maternal circulation was described in the 90s. The formation and transport of placental debris, first attributed to placental ischaemia, is at present mainly ascribed to mechanical damage caused by jet-like spurs of blood flowing into the villous space from a non-transformed spiral artery. Placental ischaemia is now restricted to the territory distal to a stenosis caused by acute atherosis–fibrinoid necrosis and lipid accumulation—and to vasoconstriction of the spiral arteries that have maintained smooth muscle cells.

The components of placental shedding trigger significant inflammation that leads to endothelial dysfunction, vasoconstriction, hyperpermeability, platelet aggregation, and glomerular endothelial swelling.

Among the soluble factors, the most prominent is soluble receptor 1 of VEGF (sFLT-1 VEGF) (which traps VEGF and its homologue placental growth factor (PlGF)), soluble endoglin, agonistic antibodies that bind to angiotensin receptor 1, reactive oxygen species, and cytokines.

Early onset preeclampsia

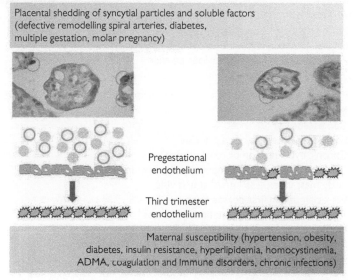

Figure 21.1 Diagram depicting the main mechanisms leading to generalized endothelial dysfunction that constitutes the clinical expression of pre-eclampsia, placental shedding of syncytial particles and soluble factors, or an underlying dysfunction, either alone or in varying combinations. Micrographs show placental villi with syncytial protrusions that precede their deportation (empty circles); these and soluble factors (full circles) enter the maternal circulation and activate endothelial cells (spiked borders).

Clinical systemic expression of endothelial damage may be secondary solely to placental shedding and leads to early-onset PE, to pre-existing maternal dysfunction which expresses in late-onset PE, or to combinations of both factors which dysregulate the maternal–placental equilibrium (Figure 21.1). In any case, it is tantamount to regarding antihypertensive treatment as a correction of an epiphenomenon.

21.3.3 Predictors of pre-eclampsia

No predictive biomarker has yet been incorporated into general obstetric practice. However, several conditions increase its probability (Box 21.1). Curiously, smoking represents a protective factor but is associated with low-weight infants.

Increased resistance and pulse pressure of uterine arteries—that reflect impaired transformation of the uterine spiral arteries—can be detected at around the 20th gestational week.

Box 21.1 Factors that predispose to pre-eclampsia–eclampsia

Associated with the couple
- Nulliparity*/primipaternity
- Limited previous exposure to paternal sperms
- Pre-eclampsia in father's previous partner

Associated with the mother
- Previous pre-eclampsia, hypertensive disorders of pregnancy, or intrauterine growth restriction, stillbirth**
- Adolescence or advanced age*
- Long interval between pregnancies*
- Chronic hypertension or renal disease**
- Coagulation disorders (antiphospholipid syndrome, lupus)**
- Body mass index ≥35 kg/m² at first visit
- Pre-eclampsia in first-degree relatives*
- Type 1 and 2 diabetes, gestational diabetes**
- Insulin resistance
- Office blood pressure between 135–139 and 80–89 mmHg at booking
- Two previous miscarriages
- Early cardiovascular disease in mother, father, or siblings (<65 years in women, <60 years in men)
- Surreptitious infections

Exogenous factors
- Malnutrition
- Stress

Associated with pregnancy
- Altered Doppler at 11–13 weeks**
- Multiple gestation**
- Assisted reproduction
- Molar pregnancy
- Fetal hydrops
- Structural or genetic congenital defects (T13, triploidy)

* Low-dose aspirin with >1 risk factor.
** Low-dose aspirin with one risk factor.

21.3.4 Prevention of pre-eclampsia

21.3.4.1 Aspirin

The Collaborative Low-dose Aspirin Study in Pregnancy showed a reduction of severe and early-onset PE. Best prevention of PE, severe PE, and intrauterine growth restriction has been observed when aspirin is started at ≤16 weeks when remodelling of the spiral arteries is still incomplete. Aspirin has not been associated with maternal or newborn haemorrhages and has been shown to be innocuous in offsprings at 12 and 18 months. Recommended doses of between 75 and 150 mg/day should be maintained up to 36–37 weeks.

21.3.4.2 Calcium supplementation

Various evidences have shown an inverse relationship between calcium intake and gestational hypertension, the incidence of PE, and preterm birth. These support supplementation with 1.2–2.5 g/day in women who present with a nutritional deficiency and an estimated low calcium intake.

21.3.4.3 L-arginine supplementation

Prolonged oral administration of the substrate of nitric oxide (6.6 g/day or 1 g/10 kg) to women at risk of PE, gestational hypertension, or chronic hypertension reduces blood pressure, the incidence of PE, preterm birth, and pulsatility indices of the umbilical artery, and increases urinary nitrites, pulsatility of the cerebral artery, fetal weight and birthweight, and the Apgar score.

21.3.4.4 Aerobic exercise

Aerobic exercise of 35–90 minutes 3–4 times a week in singleton and uncomplicated pregnancy is associated with increased vaginal deliveries, reduction of diabetes, and gestational hypertension, without modifying the time of parturition.

21.3.4.5 Other indications

Since no evidence supports that sodium restriction or diuretics reduce the risk of PE, their use is only justified in patients with congestive cardiac failure. Rest in lateral recumbency has not proven effective. Though antioxidant vitamins reduce the risk of PE, newborns to mothers with gestational hypertension or PE have lower birthweight.

The potential benefits of pravastatin in animal models and hypertensive women deserve to be followed.

21.4 Evaluation of the hypertensive pregnant woman

21.4.1 Diagnosing hypertension in the pregnant woman

Blood pressure is measured as discussed in Chapter 4. Hypertension in pregnancy is defined as office values of ≥140/90 mmHg. Home blood pressures should be determined with devices validated in pregnancy and normal limits have to be changed to 135/85 mmHg. For ambulatory blood pressure monitoring, the limits must be set according to the gestational stage (128/82 mmHg between 9 and 16 weeks, 128/80 mmHg between 16 and 24 weeks, 132/85 mmHg between 26 and 32 weeks, and 134/86 mmHg at >33–40 weeks; the nocturnal dip fluctuates between 14–17 and 15–18 mmHg).

After a diagnosis of hypertension is established, the clinical workup is directed towards evaluating the severity of the hypertensive syndrome and identifying its type, target organ damage induced by hypertension, and the state of the fetoplacental unit. This includes a detailed clinical history, physical examination, and laboratory investigations, as discussed in Chapters 3 and 4.

In addition, there are a few aspects that are peculiar to pregnancy. The history should include maternal detection and quantification of fetal movements, which is a valuable indication of fetal health. Physical examination should include the level of conciousness, the presence of a third or fourth cardiac sound, increased epigastric sensitivity and tenderness, and a hyperactive patellar reflex. Greater vascular permeability—first recognized by increased weight—presents as facial, hand, and lumbosacral oedema. Oedema of lower extremities on its own, is frequently observed in normal pregnancies.

21.4.1.1 Laboratory investigations

It is crucial to have an early panel of investigations for pregnant women with risk factors for PE in order to enable the detection of small variations within a range of normal values.

Proteinuria of ≥300 mg/day, or a protein:creatinine ratio in an single sample of ≥300 mg/g can provide a rapid diagnosis. In terms of a dipstick test, a reading of 1 "1+" is roughly equivalent to 300 mg/24 hours. In normal gestation, serum creatinine values are low and small increases may not be recognized; thus, renal function should be evaluated by creatinine clearance. Decreased renal function and proteinuria could be due to chronic renal disease and a urine microscopic examination is mandatory.

An elevated haematocrit suggests sleep apnoea, failure of volume expansion, volume contraction due to vasoconstriction, or increased vascular permeability. Crenocytes, schistocytes esquistocytes, or low platelet count reflect severe endotelial dysfunction. A serum uric acid level of >5 mg/dL, as well as PlGF levels, is helpful to differentiate between pure gestational or chronic hypertension from superimposed PE. Hepatic enzymes reflect haemolysis and hepatocellular damage. Ventricular hypertrophy on electrocardiography or echocardiography indicates preconception hypertension.

21.4.1.2 Fetal and uterine examination

Fetal and uterine examination evaluates fetal vitality, presentation, the relationship between gestational age and uterine height, and the maturity of the cervix.

21.4.1.3 Ultrasonography and Doppler

These enable evaluation of fetal well-being, fetal growth, fetal anomalies, and abnormal haemodynamics, as well the pattern and resistance of uterine artery flow. An abnormal Doppler between 16 and 24 weeks is a sensitive predictor of PE presenting at ≤37 weeks.

21.4.1.4 Cardiotocography

This evaluates the variation in the fetal heart rate and its tolerance to contractions.

21.4.2 Management of hypertensive pregnancy

With the exception of interrupting the pregnancy and delivering the placenta, there is no treament for PE. In clinical practice, in many cases, it is necessary to prolong pregnancy in order to ensure viability of the newborn. This 'treatment' must not impair the placental circulation and enable expectant management without fetal or maternal complications, with fine titration of antihypertensives. The fact that the two patients involved may react discordantly to blood pressure variations should always be kept in mind. It is necessary to involve a neonatologist when considering interruption of pregnancy. If the gestational age is <34 weeks, induction of fetal lung maturity with two doses of steroids, 24 hours apart, is indicated. When referring to a tertiary centre with an experienced neonatal intensive care unit, it is safer to transfer the pregnant mother than a frail newborn baby.

After parturition, a placental biopsy is required in early-onset PE associated with intrauterine growth restriction and stillbirth to detect thrombi leading to procoagulant conditions and genotypes.

Since eclampsia can present up to 7 days post-partum, maternal monitoring should be continued in patients who present with postpartum PE or in whom severe PE has not been controlled 72–96 hours after delivery. A uterine ultrasound is needed to identify and extract placental residues.

21.4.3 Management of the HELLP syndrome

Maternal and fetal complications are primarily related to bleeding and the gestational age at delivery, respectively. Steroids reduce maternal and neonatal morbimortality, and increase platelets and birthweight. The most important complication of HELLP is hepatic rupture, which presents with intense and persistent epigastric pain, occasional shoulder pain, and even shock, and is associated with 50% maternal and fetal mortality. Emergency surgery is indicated when a ruptured haematoma is detected by ultrasound or CT scanning and is associated with haemodynamic instability. Expectant management can be followed for subcapsular haematomas.

21.4.4 Management of eclampsia

In most cases, convulsions are preceded by premonitory symptoms that includes neurological manifestations, such as intense headaches, hypoacusis, tinnitus, hyperreflexia or extension of the reflex area, diplopia, scotomas, blurred vision, or blindness, as well as tachycardia, fever, nausea, vomiting, epigastric pain, haematemesis, haematuria, and oliguria/anuria. In approximately 20% of cases, convulsions represent the first sign of loss of autoregulatory capacity, breakdown of the blood–brain barrier, and endothelial dysfunction. Immediate causes of death are pulmonary oedema, stroke, shock due to placental abruption, intravascular coagulation, cardiac arrest, and severe acid–base disequilibrium. Late causes of death are aspiration pneumonia and renal and hepatic failure. Eclampsia cannot be regarded as a transient and reversible event as it may have serious life-long consequences.

21.5 Antihypertensives

A study comparing tight versus less tight blood pressure control favours tight control and recommends reductions of blood pressure to attain a systolic blood pressure of <160 mmHg and a diastolic blood pressure of 85 mmHg. Blood pressure-lowering drugs must reduce maternal blood pressure without concomitantly reducing uterine perfusion, interfering with fetal development and adaptation mechanisms, or modifying laboratory investigations necessary for follow-up.

21.5.1 Oral antihypertensives for maintenance treatment of hypertensive disorders of pregnancy

- Methyldopa: an old antihypertensive now reserved for gestation. It has a wide dose range and thus allows slow titration. Offspring followed up for 7 years presented with sleep pattern disorders.
- Labetalol: an effective antihypertensive with no relevant effects on the mother. Offspring followed up for 7 years showed an increased risk of attention-deficit/hyperactivity disorder.
- Hydralazine: may cause headache but does not increase the basally higher maternal heart rate.
- Calcium antagonists: effective antihypertensives that do not affect uteroplacental perfusion. Potentiation of calcium antagonists and magnesium is anecdotal and does not preclude use of the combination.

21.5.2 Antihypertensives for emergency treatment of hypertensive disorders of pregnancy

If a rapid fall in blood pressure is required, parenteral antihypertensives should be administered, with the sole exception of nifedipine capsules.

- Nifedipine: though use of capsules is contraindicated in the management of other hypertensive crises, they represent a valuable tool in gestation. Capsules can be punctured in order to deliver sublingual drops that allow precise titration (1 drop is equivalent to 1 mg). As it reduces uterine contractility, it may prolong labour.
- Labetalol: can be administrated by infusion or intravenous boluses.
- Hydralazine: can be administered intravenously or intramuscularly.
- Diuretics: use of potent and rapidly active furosemide is limited to hypertensive emergencies, including pulmonary oedema. Due to elevated

aldosterone levels in pregnancy, plasma potassium levels should be monitored and hypokalaemia corrected to prevent arrhythmias provoked by eventual anaesthesia.

21.5.3 Antihypertensives contraindicated in pregnancy

Blockade of the renin–angiotensin system (RAS) by angiotensin I-converting enzyme inhibitors (ACEIs) and angiotensin II receptor antagonists (ARA2) is absolutely contraindicated in gestation. As these represent the first-line antihypertensives for treatment of essential hypertension in young patients, it is highly possible that many women of childbearing age are exposed to them. Their use in the first trimester increases the risk of abortion but does not affect the fetus after discontinuation. ACEIs and ARA2 should only be indicated for young women who use effective contraceptive methods because they reduce placental flow and cause oligoamnios, renal impairment, stillbirth, and low birthweight. Moreover, so far, cranial defects in more than 13 babies have been reported. The only indication related to pregnancy is maintenance of preconception blockade of the RAS for 1–2 years in order to reduce arterial stiffness which, at the level of the spiral arteries, could facilitate trophoblast invasion.

Atenolol reduces placental perfusion and fetal weight, and provokes bradycardia in the newborn. Spironolactone may feminize a male fetus.

21.5.4 Magnesium sulphate for preventing and managing eclampsia

Between 1995 and 2002, the Eclampsia and the Magpie Trial demonstrated that magnesium sulphate reduces the risk of eclampsia and has a protective effect in terms of maternal vasospasm, the fetal central neural system, and placental abruption. Diazepam and phenytoin are usually limited to patients with contraindications to magnesium sulphate, such as myasthenia gravis and myocardial ischaemia or infarction. If magnesium sulphate infusion is run over 5 days, neonatal hypermagnesaemia, hypocalcaemia, and skeletal defects should be monitored for.

21.6 Aetiologies of chronic hypertension in pregnancy

21.6.1 Essential hypertension

Twenty-five per cent of patients with HDP have chronic hypertension, and as in the general population, most of these patients are diagnosed with essential hypertension. Many women do not have a pre-gestational diagnosis of hypertension and often hypertension is diagnosed during obstetric assessments, making it impossible to determine the duration of hypertension. In the majority of women, a small reduction in blood pressure is observed between 10 and 25 weeks, which may allow a transient reduction or discontinuation of antihypertensive medications.

If a hypertensive woman does not achieve good preconception blood pressure control, or she presents with decreased renal function, her chances of having a successful pregnancy are limited; thus, if she gets pregnant, it is important that her management is shared between the obstetrician and internist. In addition to routine assessment for proteinuria, creatinine clearance, serum uric acid, liver enzymes, and platelet counts should also be included in order to detect super-imposed PE. Monitoring of the fetus and uterine artery blood flow should be performed at shorter intervals.

Perinatal outcome can be improved by interrupting pregnancy between 37 and 38 weeks. Oxytocin can be used to induce labour despite its mild hypertensive effect. Use of non-steroidal anti-inflammatory agents should be restricted and ergot derivatives are contraindicated.

21.6.2 Secondary arterial hypertension

All patients with secondary hypertension should be followed up in tertiary centres that have high-risk specialist obstetric units that have experience in the complex diagnostic and management aspects of this condition.

Chronic renal diseases affect maternal and fetal outcomes, even if renal function is mildly decreased. When renal function is markedly reduced pre-gestationally or deteriorates during pregnancy, initiation of haemodialysis is indicated.

- Renovascular stenosis: due to the predominance of fibrous lesions in young women, assessment for renovascular stenosis is recommended when hypertension cannot be managed. Hypertension may have an ac-celerated course or be associated with superimposed early and severe PE. In addition, the increased diameter of aneurysmal lesions may lead to rupture. Doppler study of renal arteries during the first trimester usu-ally provides well-defined images; from the second trimester onwards, magnetic resonance imaging (MRI) without gadolinium can be performed. Angioplasty has been performed successfully in the second trimester, with shielding of the fetus.

- Primary hyperaldosteronism: patients with a pre-gestational diagnosis may have their blood pressure lowered and hypokalaemia corrected since high progesterone levels antagonize the effects of aldosterone. Chronic hypertension that improves with pregnancy and presents with an abrupt increase in blood pressure in the post-partum period should prompt as-sessment for primary aldosteronism. During gestation, a differential diag-nosis of primary aldosteronism cannot be performed due to the effects of progesterone and gestational changes in the renin–angiotensin–aldos-terone system. Amiloride (a potassium-sparing diuretic), methyldopa, or calcium channel antagonists are recommended to control hyperten-sion, the most critical goal of management. If blood pressure is hard to control, an adenoma identified on nuclear MRI may be resected through laparoscopy. Post-partum increase in blood pressure can be minimized curtailed by limiting use of sodium and non-steroidal analgesic agents and avoiding ergotamine derivatives.

- Aortic coarctation: This can be diagnosed during physical examination. It is associated with miscarriages, gestational hypertension, and fetal cardiac defects in up to 3% of cases. On the other hand, blood pressure can be easily controlled and PE is absent. Pregnancy may increase the gradient of a native or restenosed coarctation by morphological changes to the aortic wall. In order to lower the risk of aortic dissection or rupture, it is necessary to reduce left ventricular contraction and maintain blood pressure to below 130/80 mmHg, whilst monitoring fetal weight and uterine artery blood flow.

- Phaeochromocytoma: this represents an infrequent cause of hypertension but should be diagnosed due to high maternal and fetal mortality associated with undiagnosed cases and due to changes in blood pressure during labour or a Caesarean section provoked by pressure on the tumoural mass. It must be suspected when a patient with stable hypertension has paroxysmal rises in blood pressure that is accompanied by a sudden onset of intense headache, profuse sweating, tachycardia, arrhythmia, episodic hypotension, heat intolerance, behavioural changes, constipation, and weight reduction. Plasma or urinary levels of catecholamines or metanephrines confirm the diagnosis, but these results can be influenced by the use of methyldopa and labetalol. The patient should be managed in a highly specialized centre for accurate diagnosis, tumour identification and location and blood pressure management. The treatment options generally includes tumour resection up to the 24th gestational week or for medical treatment thereafter, with fine blood pressure control with alpha and beta blockade once fetal lung maturity is achieved. Tumor resection can be performed after a Caesarean section or in the post-partum period if the decision for medical therapy was made during pregnancy.

21.7 Post-partum management of hypertensive pregnancies

21.7.1 Early post-partum period

Antihypertensives usually allow progressive reduction of labour. Sodium restriction can be initiated and non-steroidal analgesics must be avoided.

There have been a few reports on the safety of antihypertensive drugs in breastfeeding. Beta blockers with a high protein binding are recommended (propranolol, oxprenolol, dilevalol, mepindolol) as compared to those with a low binding (atenolol, metoprolol, nadolol, acebutolol, sotalol). Methyldopa is minimally excreted in milk and has no effects on the baby. Nitrendipine and nimodipine have minimal excretion, whilst verapamil is variably excreted. Captopril and enalapril have minimal excretion but should be avoided in premature babies. Caution should be exerted with diuretics as they can cause water and electrolyte disturbances in the neonate.

21.7.2 Long-term maternal follow-up

Since Jonsdottir et al. communicated in 1995 that the relative risk of dying from ischaemic heart disease was 1.9- and 2.6-fold in pre-eclamptic and eclamptic women, respectively, numerous other long-term follow-up studies have corroborated these findings of an association between hypertensive pregnancy with the risk of cardiovascular diseases. Four systematic reviews and meta-analyses have provided concordant relative risks of PE with hypertension, cardiovascular disease, ischaemic heart disease, stroke, and cardiovascular death (Table 21.2). The risk also correlates with the severity of maternal and neonatal complications such as recurrent PE, intrauterine growth retardation, and preterm birth.

Unfortunately, screening for cardiovascular risks has not been incorporated into pre-, intra-, and post-gestational follow-up, in order to correct modifiable factors. It is feasible to postulate that post-partum modification of cardiovascular risks could improve the outcome of future pregnancies, but no reports are currently available.

The reproductive history is not a component of routine evaluation of women who present with angina, despite the American Heart Association highlighting in 2011 the remote risk of adverse obstetric outcomes with cardiac ischaemic disease, the leading cause of death. Undoubtedly, identification of poor obstetric outcomes could improve detection of myocardial ischaemia in women, who are

Table 21.2 relative risk and 95% confidence intervals associated with pre-eclampsia

	Bellamy et al., 2007	McDonald et al., 2008	Brown, 2013	Wu et al., 2017
Hypertension	3.70 (2.70–5.05)		3.30 (2.51–3.89)	
Cardiovascular disease		2.48 (1.22–5.90)	2.28 (1.87–2.39)	
Fatal/non-fatal myocardial ischaemia	2.16 (1.86–2.52)			2.50 (1.43–4.37)
Stroke	1.81 (1.45–2.27)	2.03 (1.95–263)	1.77 (1.43–4.37)	1.81 (1.29–2.55)
Cardiovascular death		2.29 (1.73–3.04)		2.21 (1.83–2.66)

more likely than men to have an atypical presentation, undergo less non-invasive and invasive testing, and be undertreated as they have more frequently non-obstructed coronary arteries, but with microvascular dysfunction and reduced coronary reserve.

21.7.3 Long-term control of offspring from a hypertensive pregnancy

Gestational hypertension causes preterm birth and low birthweight. Barker in 1989 associated lower birthweight with higher blood pressures in childhood and higher cardiovascular mortality in adults, and postulated that adult diseases initiate in fetal life. This concept has been extended to different chronic illnesses in adulthood that involve diverse systems and are caused by genotypic variations, epigenetic changes, and environmental intra- and extrauterine factors; with respect to the latter, a mismatch between fetal and postnatal life exacerbates the intrauterine damage.

From the hypertension perspective, it is highly probable that pressor mechanisms are stimulated in the fetus in order to protect their cerebral perfusion, resulting in early changes to their arterial morphology. Renal development may be also affected by low birthweight (<2500 g) and prematurity (<37 weeks), causing a reduction in number of renal glomeruli that stresses the remaining glomeruli. This results in reduced sodium excretion and secondary focal segmental glomerulosclerosis, which then further evolves to progressive renal failure. This evolution can be prevented by early strict blood pressure control with RAS blockade, which also decreases intraglomerular hypertension.

21.8 Conclusion

Identification of risk factors for HDP, precise, timely, and simultaneous management, and early identification of long-term risks of mother and offspring amplify the responsibility of the obstetric team at the individual and epidemiological levels.

KEY REFERENCES

Brown MA, Magee LA, Kenny LC, et al. (2018). Hypertensive disorders of pregnancy: ISSHP classification, diagnosis and management recommendations for international practice. *Hypertension* 72:24–43.

Burton GJ, Redman CW, Roberts JM, Moffett A (2019). Pre-eclampsia: pathophysiology and clinical implications. *BMJ* 366:l2381.

Cífková R, Johnson MR, Kahan T, et al. (2019). Peripartum management of hypertension: a position paper of the ESC Council on Hypertension and the European Society of Hypertension. *Eur Heart J Cardiovasc Pharmacother* 6:384–93.

Duckitt K, Harrington D (2005). Risk factors for pre-eclampsia at antenatal booking: systematic review of controlled studies. *BMJ* 33:565–72.

Huppertz B (2018). The critical role of trophoblast development in the etiology of preeclampsia. *Curr Pharm Biotechnol* **19**:771–80.

Levine RJ, Maynard SE, Qian C, et al. (2004). Circulating angiogenic factors and the risk of preeclampsia. *N Engl J Med* **350**:672–83.

National Institute for Health and Care Excellence (2019). Hypertension in pregnancy: diagnosis and management. Available from: https://www.nice.org.UK/guidance/ng133

Quesada O, Shufelt C, Bairey Merz CN (2020). Can we improve cardiovascular disease for women using data under our noses? A need for changes in policy and focus. *JAMA Cardiol* **5**:1398–400.

Romundstad PR, Magnussen E, Smith GD, Vatten LJ (2010). Hypertension in pregnancy and later cardiovascular risk. Common antecedents? *Circulation* **122**:579–84.

Søndergaard MM, Hlatky MA, Stefanick ML, et al. (2020). Association of adverse pregnancy outcomes with risk of atherosclerotic cardiovascular disease in postmenopausal women. *JAMA Cardiol* **5**:1390–8.

Valdés G (2017). Preeclampsia and cardiovascular disease: interconnected paths that enable detection of the subclinical stages of obstetric and cardiovascular diseases. *Integr Blood Press Control* **10**:17–23.

CHAPTER 21

CHAPTER 22

Hypertensive emergencies

Alena Shantsila

KEY POINTS

- A hypertensive emergency is a severe form of hypertension that causes acute organ damage, which therefore requires blood pressure lowering in hospital settings.
- Target organ damage includes hypertensive encephalopathy, retinal lesions, pre-eclampsia and eclampsia, acute left ventricular failure with pulmonary oedema, coronary ischaemia, acute aortic dissection, and renal failure.
- The target blood pressure to reach is dictated by clinical features. Typically, titratable parenteral drugs are used to avoid a sudden blood pressure drop, as this could result in ischaemic complications.
- Such patients are referred for antihypertensive management optimization and exclusion of possible secondary causes of hypertension.

22.1 Introduction

Hypertensive emergencies are a group of acute conditions, defined by the presence of severe hypertension (usually in excess of 180/110 mmHg) associated with acute hypertension-mediated organ damage. Organs which can be damaged are the heart, brain, retina, kidneys, and large arteries. This acute damage is, in most cases, life-threatening, requiring immediate hospital admission to administer blood pressure-lowering therapy in a carefully controlled manner. Data show that it is not only the absolute value of blood pressure increase, but also the rate and level of elevation that determine the extent of acute organ damage.

Acute severe elevation of blood pressure above 180/110 mmHg in the absence of acute end-organ damage is referred to as hypertensive urgency. The key difference with emergencies is that absence of life-threatening complications means that hospital admission is not indicated. Use of oral antihypertensive medications is recommended as intravenous therapy does not improve cardiovascular outcomes.

According to the 2018 European Society of Hypertension Position Document on management of hypertensive emergencies, the most common clinical features of hypertensive emergencies are malignant hypertension with or without acute renal failure, coronary ischaemia or acute cardiogenic pulmonary oedema, acute stroke or hypertensive encephalopathy, acute aortic disease (aneurysm or dissection), and eclampsia or severe pre eclampsia. These clinical features are key in determining the three main components of the therapeutic plan: (1) timeline and safe target blood pressure; (2) choice of intravenous drug therapy; and (3) choice of other treatments if required.

22.2 Epidemiological aspects

In general, the proportion of emergency department presentations with hypertensive emergencies is 1 in every 200 patients. Hypertensive emergencies most commonly occur in patients known to have hypertension and is usually due to inadequate management, reflecting the problem of medication non-adherence and/or limited access to healthcare. However, some patients might present *de novo*, with no prior documentation of hypertension. The leading causes of an acute hypertensive emergency presentation in the United States are heart failure, stroke, and myocardial infarction, followed by intracranial haemorrhage and aortic dissection. There are several reassuring data showing that in-hospital mortality has improved significantly in the last decade, with 50% risk reduction from 2002 till 2012. Patients who survive a hypertension emergency remain at higher risk of intermediate mortality, compared to hypertensives with no hospital admission.

22.3 Pathophysiology

The key pathophysiological mechanism of hypertensive emergencies is an intense increase in systemic vascular resistance, leading to blood pressure elevation (Figure 22.1). Blood pressure elevation increases vascular wall mechanical stress and causes endothelial dysfunction. Failure of autoregulatory processes to compensate leads to increased vascular wall permeability, oedema, coagulation cascade and platelet activation, development of macroangiopathic haemolytic anaemia, fibrinoid necrosis of arterioles, and further microcirculatory damage. The renin–angiotensin system is activated and pressure natriuresis further stimulates the activation. All of the above processes can manifest in target organ ischaemia and relevant clinical presentations.

22.4 Clinical features of hypertensive emergencies

22.4.1 Malignant hypertension

Malignant phase hypertension is a hypertensive emergency characterized by severe elevation in systolic blood pressure and out-of-range diastolic blood pressure and advanced retinopathy, defined as bilateral flame-shaped haemorrhages, cotton-wool spots, and/or papilloedema (Figure 22.2). Over the 24 years of the West Birmingham Malignant Hypertension Registry, the average level of systolic and diastolic blood pressures at presentation has remained surprisingly unchanged (average 228/142 mmHg). It is important to emphasize that diastolic

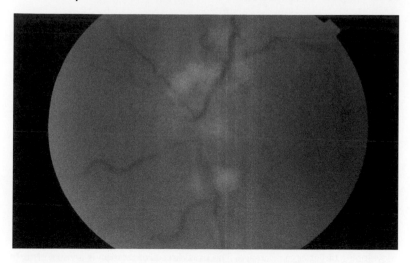

Figure 22.1 Ocular fundus in malignant hypertension showing cotton wool spots, haemorrhages, and papilloedema.

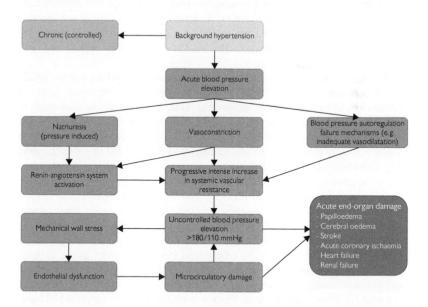

Figure 22.2 Main pathophysiological mechanisms of hypertensive emergencies.

CHAPTER 22

blood pressure >120 mmHg should not be used as a rigid criterion for diagnosis. Similarly, typical eye changes might also be absent in some patients. In fact, it has recently been suggested that malignant hypertension should be reclassified to hypertension with multiorgan damage and new diagnostic criteria of impairment of at least three different target organs (kidney, heart, brain, microangiopathy) added.

The main histological feature of malignant hypertension is fibrinoid necrosis of arterioles in various tissues, including the kidney. This could be accompanied by mucoid intimal proliferation in renal interlobular arteries and ischaemic dysfunction of the glomerular tufts. These changes trigger marked activation of the renin–angiotensin system, systemic vasoconstriction, and progression of hypertension. Usually, plasma renin activity and aldosterone levels are much higher in these patients than in severe hypertension, despite quite comparable blood pressure values.

Malignant hypertension is commonly underdiagnosed and up to 75% of patients with malignant hypertension would only be seen the first time, after developing target organ damage. The usual first presentation is a visual disturbance (acute or subacute) that may be accompanied by a headache. The presence of these symptoms should always be treated with a suspicion of possible malignant hypertension. In 10–15% of cases, the first presentation is hypertensive encephalopathy, and in some cases, acute renal failure is the first presentation. In the emergency department setting, fundoscopy is required, as well as urinalysis, blood urea and electrolytes, full blood count, 12-lead electrocardiogram (ECG), and transthoracic echocardiography, and computed tomography (CT) of the head if indicated.

Progressive decline in renal function to end-stage renal failure is still a significant threat. Long-term optimal blood pressure control is an important factor to preserve renal function, as end-stage renal disease is a major cause of death in patients with malignant hypertension. Long-term survival of patients with malignant hypertension has improved dramatically. There has been an improvement in 5-year mortality from 76% for patients diagnosed before 1967 to 7% for patients diagnosed between 1997 and 2011.

During admission in the emergency department, in the absence of hypertensive encephalopathy, elevated blood pressure in patients with malignant hypertension needs to be reduced within several hours (Table 22.1). The target mean arterial pressure is a reduction by 20–25% from the presenting values. Recommended first-line medications are intravenous labetalol and nicardipine. An alternative option is urapidil. It needs to be emphasized that in the acute phase, patients with malignant hypertension are often volume-depleted. This is why use of angiotensin-converting enzyme (ACE) inhibitors, even in low doses, can result in a massive blood pressure drop. Volume depletion must be corrected by intravenous saline infusion in such cases.

Hospital discharge must be followed by regular follow-up, which should be at least monthly at the beginning. Follow-up visits with the responsible physician

Table 22.1 Management of hypertensive emergencies in hospital settings

Clinical features	Timeline and target BP	First-line treatment	Second-line treatment
Malignant hypertension	Several hours to reduce MAP by 20–25%	Labetalol, nicardipine	Nitroprusside, urapidil
Hypertensive encephalopathy	Immediately to reduce MAP by 20–25%	Labetalol, nicardipine	Nitroprusside
Eclampsia and severe pre-eclampsia	Immediately to below 160/105 mmHg	Labetalol or nicardipine and magnesium	
Acute stroke			
Ischaemic and SBP >220 mmHg or DBP >120 mmHg	Within 1 hour to reduce MAP by 15%	Labetalol, nicardipine	Nitroprusside
Ischaemic for thrombolysis and SBP >185 mmHg or DBP >110 mmHg	Within 1 hour to reduce MAP by 15%	Labetalol, nicardipine	Nitroprusside
Haemorrhagic and SBP >180 mmHg	Immediately to SBP below 130 mmHg	Labetalol, nicardipine	Urapidil
Acute coronary event	Immediately to SBP below 140 mmHg	Nitroglycerine, labetalol	Urapidil
Acute cardiogenic pulmonary oedema	Immediately to SBP below 140 mmHg	Nitroprusside or nitroglycerine with loop diuretic	Urapidil with loop diuretic
Acute aortic disease	Immediately to SBP below 120 mmHg and HR below 60 beats/min	Esmolol and nitroprusside or nitroglycerine or nicardipine	Labetalol or metoprolol

BP, blood pressure; DBP, diastolic blood pressure; MAP, mean arterial pressure; SBP, systolic blood pressure; HR, heart rate.

are to optimize antihypertensive medications and to investigate for possible secondary causes of hypertension.

22.4.2 Hypertensive encephalopathy or acute stroke

Patients with hypertensive encephalopathy present with sudden onset of headache, nausea, and vomiting, accompanied by visual disturbances or field loss.

Neurological symptoms of confusion and drowsiness might progress further if blood pressure is not reduced, leading to seizures and coma.

Past medical history often reveals discontinuation, typically sudden, of antihypertensive treatment or inadequate treatment. Failure of cerebral autoregulatory vasoconstriction, in response to a sudden blood pressure rise, results in arteriolar dilatation and vascular dysfunction. Following this, the brain becomes hyperperfused, with accompanying impairment of the blood–brain barrier and development of cerebral oedema. The prevalence of this complication is now low; however, a retrospective analysis of data from the United States showed an increasing trend in hospital admissions of patients with either hypertensive encephalopathy or malignant hypertension since 2007. This observation could reflect improved recognition and diagnoses of malignant hypertension with encephalopathy, as admissions for essential hypertension fall. In patients with hypertensive encephalopathy, the typical finding on CT or magnetic resonance imaging (MRI) is white matter oedema, which is reversible following blood pressure stabilization. Either of these scans is essential for ruling out the differential diagnosis of cerebral infarction and haemorrhages.

Blood pressure-lowering treatment needs to be initiated immediately, with the target to reduce mean arterial pressure by 20–25% initially. The preferred pharmacological option in this situation is parenteral labetalol, due to its protective effect on cerebral blood flow, following blood pressure reduction. Sodium nitroprusside and nitrates have also been used successfully and are recommended. If a hypertension-associated seizure occurs during or immediately after pregnancy as consistent with eclampsia, the symptoms are often very similar and treatment options are parenteral labetalol, magnesium sulphate, and considerations for early fetal delivery.

In patients admitted following any acute stroke, modest elevation in blood pressure is a compensatory mechanism due to cerebral blood flow being pressure-dependent. That is why any excessive blood pressure reduction may intensify risk of further infarction and/or haemorrhage and is associated with negative long-term neurological outcomes. Currently, blood pressure lowering in acute ischaemic stroke is recommended if it is very high (above 220/120 mmHg) or if the patient is considered for thrombolytic therapy, or if the patient develops other complications (acute coronary syndrome, heart failure, or aortic dissection). In these cases, the aim is to reduce mean arterial pressure by 15% within 1 hour. For haemorrhagic stroke, the threshold for blood pressure lowering is systolic blood pressure above 180 mmHg. The preferred and currently recommended first-line medications are again labetalol and nicardipine. Several randomized clinical trials failed to confirm the benefit of intensive blood pressure lowering to values of <140/90 mmHg for survival and improved neurological outcomes over early and later recovery periods. Data from the large Safe Implementation of Thrombolysis in Stroke International Stroke Thrombolysis Register (SITS-ISTR) showed a U-shaped relationship of death and physical independence with systolic blood pressure, and it appears that systolic blood pressure of 141–150 mmHg is associated with the most favourable outcome.

22.4.3 Coronary ischaemia or acute cardiogenic pulmonary oedema

In patients with hypertensive emergencies complicated by acute coronary syndrome and chest pain (unstable angina or acute myocardial infarction), prompt reduction of cardiac afterload by an appropriate decrease in blood pressure can improve coronary perfusion. This needs to be done without a compensatory increase in heart rate, as otherwise, a reduction in diastolic filling time may minimize the expected haemodynamic benefits. The goal is to decrease systolic blood pressure below 140 mmHg in a controlled manner, with care to avoid further myocardial or brain ischaemia. This goal should be achieved by initiation of intravenous nitrates and a beta blocker (labetalol). If significant tachycardia is present, high doses of beta blockers may be required. An alternative second-line treatment with urapidil can also be considered. The risk of bleeding due to use of anticoagulation or antithrombotic therapy should also be carefully considered. Although prompt antiplatelet therapy is typically given in acute coronary syndrome, if there is a clear primary hypertensive emergency complicated by angina, priority should be given to blood pressure reduction. It is not recommended to use sodium nitroprusside in such situations as it reduces coronary blood flow in the presence of coronary stenosis. Also, sublingual nifedipine is no longer recommended, as its oral absorption is not complete and later gastric absorption results in difficult-to-control hypotension (additionally, it is associated with an increase in heart rate).

Patients with pulmonary oedema secondary to hypertensive emergencies usually present with severe dyspnoea, respiratory crackles, crepitations in the lungs, and raised jugular venous pressure. A chest X-ray is the first investigation these patients would need to confirm the clinical suspicion. Transthoracic echocardiography is useful to quickly evaluate whether systolic and/or diastolic function is affected, to assess for left ventricular hypertrophy, and to evaluate aortic and mitral valve function. The main aim of treatment is to reduce cardiac pre- and afterload without affecting cardiac contractility. The blood pressure goal is the same as with acute coronary syndrome—to reduce systolic blood pressure below 140 mmHg in a controlled manner.

An infusion of nitroprusside or nitrates is the first choice, as it would reduce preload and afterload. Nitrates are also recommended, but high doses might be needed. An alternative is a second-line treatment with urapidil. Loop diuretics are also usually administered to reduce volume overload and further reduce blood pressure. Following patient stabilization and blood pressure reduction, it is important to consider the long-term use of ACE inhibitors, as they have been shown to improve long-term survival and lead to regression of left ventricular hypertrophy if present.

ACE inhibitors are best avoided in the early stage as they may, even at a very low dose, cause precipitous falls in blood pressure and life-threatening reduction of cerebral perfusion, particularly when patients are fluid-depleted due to diuretic therapy or in the presence of renal artery stenosis.

22.4.4 Acute aortic disease (aneurysm or dissection)

In patients with hypertensive emergencies and chest pain, aortic dissection should always be suspected and ruled out. Typical chest pain associated with aortic dissection is tearing pain that radiates to the back. Other clinical features suggestive of aortic dissection are asymmetry of pulses between the right and left arms, confirmed by large differences in blood pressure measured in both arms. Further diagnostic tests will have to be performed promptly to detect the vascular bed affected, which would define the management options (surgical versus non-surgical). The test of choice in suspected aortic dissection is a contrast thoracic CT or MRI. Transoesophageal echocardiography is also quite informative, but invasive, and its use is limited by the need for adequate blood pressure control before the scan. Transthoracic echocardiography has a limited role in the assessment of suspected aortic dissection due to poor pickup rates.

On suspicion of aortic dissection, the approach for blood pressure reduction is to reach the goal of a systolic blood pressure of 120 mmHg and a heart rate of 60 beats/min as soon as possible. The pathophysiological reason behind this is to reduce the aortic wall shear stress and subsequently to limit further progression and spread of the dissection. Therefore, beta blockers are the first-line treatment. Esmolol is recommended to be used with a short-acting vasodilator such as sodium nitroprusside.

22.5 Treatment

The main and most important determinant in the management plan is the target organ affected. Acute hypertension-mediated organ damage includes microangiopathy, renal failure, coronary ischaemia or cardiogenic pulmonary oedema, stroke or hypertensive encephalopathy, aortic disease, eclampsia, or severe pre-eclampsia. The most important goal is to stop and prevent further damage of the organs affected by reducing blood pressure in a strictly controlled manner. Current approaches and their pathophysiological justifications are discussed in detail in the relevant previous sections. A comprehensive summary of currently recommended treatments and blood pressure targets is provided in Table 22.1. The magnitude and speed of blood pressure reduction are driven by the clinical presentation. The most rapid reduction, to different blood pressure targets, is required in patients with acute aortic dissection, pulmonary oedema and/or coronary event, and eclampsia. The best approach to treating acute strokes in hypertensive emergencies is still a matter of debate. The recommended first-line medications in the majority of cases are intravenous labetalol and nicardipine infusions.

Following hospital discharge, patients must be referred to the responsible physician for antihypertensive medication optimization and to investigate for possible secondary causes of hypertension.

22.6 Conclusion

Hypertensive emergencies are relatively uncommon, but potentially life-threatening, conditions that need timely assessment and management. They can manifest with a range of different presentations with acute hypertension-mediated organ damage. It is important to be vigilant to the variety of such presentations and ensure a holistic approach to their management.

KEY REFERENCES

Lip GY, Beevers M, Beevers G (1994). The failure of malignant hypertension to decline: a survey of 24 years' experience in a multiracial population in England. *J Hypertens* 12:1297–305.

Shantsila A, Shantsila E, Beevers DG, Lip GYH (2017). Predictors of 5-year outcomes in malignant phase hypertension: the West Birmingham Malignant Hypertension Registry. *J Hypertens* 35:2310–14.

van den Born BH, Lip GYH, Brguljan-Hitij J, et al. (2019). ESC Council on hypertension position document on the management of hypertensive emergencies. *Eur Heart J Cardiovasc Pharmacother* 5:37–46.

Vaughan CJ, Delanty N (2000). Hypertensive emergencies. *Lancet* 356:411–17.

CHAPTER 23

Treatment of the older adult

Asangaedem Akpan

KEY POINTS

- Hypertension, especially isolated systolic hypertension, is common in older adults.
- Overtreatment can be harmful, and caution must be exercised in the very old.
- Ambulatory blood pressure monitoring (ABPM) is ideal to confirm the diagnosis of hypertension.
- Hypertension is a major risk factor for cerebrovascular accidents, coronary artery disease, heart failure, retinopathy, chronic renal disease, and cognitive impairment.
- Non-pharmacological approaches are an integral part of management.
- Management can be challenging because of side effects, polypharmacy, coexisting multiple chronic conditions, frailty, orthostatic hypotension, falls, and cognitive impairment.

23.1 Introduction

Blood pressure readings are a continuous variable in the population and follow a Gaussian distribution. It is therefore not possible to define a 'normal blood pressure' as what is considered 'normal' would vary according to age, sex, and even race. For guidelines, values above a certain threshold at which there is increased likelihood of cardiovascular risk are chosen, and treatment offered. Likewise, there is increasing evidence that below a certain threshold, there is increased risk of morbidity and mortality, especially in the very old (age 85 years and above) and those with moderate to severe frailty.

Hypertension, as defined by guidelines, is present in over two-thirds of adults aged 60 years and above. It is a major risk factor for cerebrovascular accidents, myocardial infarction, heart failure, retinopathy, chronic renal disease, and cognitive impairment. Treating hypertension in older adults has reduced morbidity and mortality.

23.2 Pathophysiology

Atherosclerosis and calcification of peripheral arteries lead to reduced arterial compliance and a rise in systolic blood pressure (SBP). The diastolic blood pressure

(DBP) tends to fall after the age of 80 and this leads to a widened pulse pressure and isolated systolic hypertension, which are considered to be independent risk factors. Diastolic hypertension accounts for <10% of cases of hypertension after the age of 70. Pulse pressure increases with age and has emerged as a significant risk factor for coronary artery disease events in older adults. Some studies have shown pulse pressure is a stronger risk factor than SBP, DBP, or mean pressure in older adults. Orthostatic or postural hypotension is more common in older people and results from a sustained drop in blood pressure on standing. Where it coexists, it can be problematic in managing hypertension.

23.3 Detection of hypertension

High blood pressure is generally considered to be asymptomatic. Headaches are attributed to the condition, but clinical studies have not proved this. It is often asymptomatic and thus has been referred to as a 'silent killer'. Blood pressure fluctuates with day-to-day activities and with various other natural life events. These fluctuations are thought to be much greater in older than in younger individuals.

Pseudohypertension refers to a falsely increased SBP. In older adults, this ranges between 1.7% and 70%, making its actual prevalence unclear. White coat hypertension is more common in older adults. Most guidelines therefore recommend ambulatory blood pressure monitoring (ABPM) to confirm the diagnosis of hypertension. If a person is unable to tolerate ABPM, a suitable alternative is home blood pressure monitoring (HBPM). Whilst using ABPM for monitoring blood pressure, it is important to ensure that at least two measurements per hour are taken during the person's usual waking hours. A minimum of 14 measurements are needed and average calculations are taken. If HBPM is used for diagnosis of hypertension, it is important to ensure that blood pressure is measured whilst the person is seated. Two consecutive measurements are taken at least 1 minute apart for each blood pressure recording. Blood pressure should be recorded twice daily for a minimum of 4 days. Ideally, two blood pressure recordings should be taken, one in the morning and one in the evening, for 7 days.

23.4 Benefits of treating hypertension in older adults

The higher the SBP or DBP in older adults, the greater the morbidity and mortality. The benefits of treating hypertension, including isolated systolic hypertension, up to the age of 80 years are clearly demonstrated. Studies such as the Systolic Hypertension in the Elderly Program (SHEP) study, the Systolic Hypertension in the Elderly: Chinese trial China (Syst-CHINA), and the Systolic Hypertension in Europe (Syst-EUR) demonstrated that reducing blood pressure in older adults with isolated systolic hypertension prevents stroke and renal failure. It is also a recognized risk factor for all types of cognitive impairment in late life and treatment can slow progression of disease. The relative risk reduction remains the same at all ages, but as the absolute risk of complications is higher among older adults, the number needed to treat is lower in older adults.

Treating a blood pressure above 160/90 mmHg is beneficial. The Hypertension in the Very Elderly Trial (HYVET) enrolled nearly 4000 patients above the age of 80 from 11 countries. The aim of the trial was to study the risks and benefits of treating these patients with a diuretic-based regime (indapamide SR) versus placebo, with addition of the angiotensin-converting enzyme (ACE) inhibitor perindopril if required. There was a reduction in morbidity and mortality from cardiovascular events, as well as in all-cause mortality. For those already on therapy, it should be reviewed, especially those who are aged 85 years and above with frailty, as SBP below 130 mmHg has been associated with morbidity and mortality. A Cochrane systematic review has shown no difference in morbidity and mortality between continuing or discontinuing antihypertensives in older adults. The evidence though for this was stated to be low and a recommendation for further research in very old adults and those with frailty and polypharmacy was recommended.

23.5 Assessment of the older hypertensive adult

It is important to involve older people in shared decision-making regarding their treatment. Finding out what matters to them, including the outcomes in which they are interested, is critical and is the first step before assessing and treating. Involving people in their care plans will improve adherence to any agreed decisions.

Malignant hypertension is rare in older adults, but the presence of bilateral haemorrhages and cotton-wool spots would be indicative of the diagnosis. Prognosis is poor; <1% survive 1 year without adequate treatment, but 80% survive if effectively treated. If readings are >180 mmHg systolic and 110 mmHg diastolic, urgent hospital admission is needed for investigation and treatment. As autoregulation of cerebral blood flow may be impaired in these patients, it is important to avoid a sudden reduction in blood pressure.

The prevalence of secondary hypertension is low in older adults, as most causes would be expected to have been detected and dealt with earlier. However, the prevalence of renovascular diseases is higher than in the younger population and may be as much as 5%. Clinical clues include abdominal bruit, peripheral vascular disease, and worsening renal function after institution of ACE inhibitors or angiotensin receptor blockers (ARBs). Other conditions such as primary aldosteronism, phaeochromocytoma, or Cushing's syndrome may occasionally be diagnosed and are potentially treatable.

23.6 Management of the older hypertensive adult

Clinical and epidemiological studies such as the Framingham Heart Study suggest that in an older adult, the SBP provides better classification and risk stratification than the DBP. The pulse pressure is marginally better than the SBP for risk stratification in this age group.

The National Institute for Health and Care Excellence (NICE) recommends a target clinic blood pressure of below 140/90 mmHg in people aged <80 years, and below 150/90 mmHg in people aged 80 years and above. The European Society of Hypertension (ESH) and the European Society of Cardiology (ESC) guidelines recommend that octogenarians with initial SBP of >160 mmHg should be treated to reduce SBP to between 150 and 140 mmHg, provided they are in good physical and mental conditions. Fit older adults under the age of 80 years should be treated in the same way as younger adults—that is, antihypertensive treatment should be considered if SBP is >140 mmHg, with a target SBP of <140 mmHg if treatment is well tolerated. When treated, the blood pressure should be lowered to a systolic value of 130–139 mmHg and a diastolic value of <80 mmHg if tolerated. Treated SBP values of <130 mmHg should be avoided. The ESC and ESH recommend all hypertensive agents can be used to treat older adults, but diuretics and calcium channel antagonists are preferred in isolated systolic hypertension.

It must be remembered that even if the target is not achieved, but blood pressure is lowered by 5–6 mmHg, it is worthwhile as this can achieve substantial cardiovascular risk reduction. Similarly, although there are no conclusive clinical trial data to suggest that treatment of stage 1 hypertension in older adults is associated with cardiovascular risk reduction, the Seventh Report of the Joint National Committee on Prevention, Detection, Evaluation, and Treatment of High Blood Pressure (JNC-7) recommends that treatment in this group should not be withheld on the basis of age alone.

23.6.1 Non-pharmacological approach

Lifestyle modifications, such as reduced salt intake to <5 g day, regular physical activity, having vegetables, fruits, and low-fat dairy products, not smoking, and not being overweight, are as important in older adults as in the rest of the population. Public health campaigns, as well as clinicians, should encourage these approaches, whilst bearing in mind that not all older people will be able to engage in all of these.

Salt reduction is important. The Trial of Non-pharmacologic Intervention in the Elderly (TONE) showed that reducing sodium to 2 g/day reduced blood pressure by 3/2 mmHg over 30 months. This drop, however, was not associated with a reduction in cardiovascular events. Nearly half of those on low-salt diet were able to discontinue their antihypertensive medications. There was a further drop in blood pressure when weight loss was combined with salt reduction.

23.6.2 Pharmacological measures

Drug therapy and non-pharmacological approaches complement each other and both are important in achieving recommended treatment targets. Recommendations on use of antihypertensive agents are similar to those for the general population. In the older adult population, the side effects of medications need to be balanced against what matters to the person receiving treatment through a shared decision-making process. This approach is more likely to result in a person taking the prescribed medications. Most older people will require at least two antihypertensives and sometimes a third is required. It is therefore important to take into consideration coexisting multiple chronic conditions and other medications that an older person may be on. Regular monitoring of side effects and drug–drug interactions is important. The different treatment groups are discussed in the respective chapters.

23.7 Specific issues in older adults

Tolerability is the main issue in treating older hypertensive adults. They are more prone to side effects. It is important to ask about side effects during each clinical encounter. Prior to prescribing and during the shared decision-making process, the more common side effects can be discussed. The individual can then pro-actively bring this to the attention of a clinician.

Older hypertensive adults can be classified into two groups; one group are those who have grown old with their hypertension and are comfortable with their medications, and the other group are those who have hypertension detected when they are old. This second group may prove difficult to manage as they may resent the lifestyle modification and medications they are required to take on. Clarifying what matters to an individual and discussing all treatment options, including the risks of non-treatment, in a supportive manner would make it easier for these changes to be accepted by an older person.

Compliance is an issue in older adults because of polypharmacy. This must be carefully considered in those with difficulty controlling their blood pressure. Compliance may be hampered by the large number of tablets that are prescribed or due to cognitive and/or physical limitations. Box 23.1 lists some of the common causes of failure of treatment in this group.

Postural hypotension is more common in older adults and can present with falls or syncope. It is recommended that blood pressure be measured in the lying and standing positions, especially if the person complains of light-headedness. If

---

Box 23.1 Possible reasons for inadequate response to treatment

- Subtherapeutic medication regime dose
- Not taking prescribed medications
- Lifestyle issues—obesity, smoking, excess alcohol intake, little or no physical activity
- Drugs used concomitantly that raise blood pressure, e.g. non-steroidal anti-inflammatory drugs, steroids
- Volume overload, e.g. high sodium intake, renal impairment
- Undetected secondary cause, e.g. phaeochromocytoma

treatment is still necessary because repeated readings suggest hypertension is still present, graduated pressure stockings to try and prevent peripheral pooling can be utilized, but it can be a difficult problem to manage.

23.8 Conclusion

Treating high blood pressure reduces morbidity and mortality. Chronological age alone should not prevent careful management of hypertension but must be balanced against overtreatment in the very old, those with moderate to severe frailty, and those with polypharmacy. Shared decision-making taking into account what matters to the person is key.

KEY REFERENCES

Akpan A, Roberts C, Bandeen-Roche K, et al. (2018). Standard set of health outcome measures for older persons. *BMC Geriatr* **18:36**–46.

Aronow WS, Fleg JL, Pepin CJ, et al.; ACCF Task Force (2011). ACCF/AHA 2011 expert consensus document on hypertension in the elderly: a report of the American College of Cardiology Foundation Task Force on Clinical Expert Consensus Documents. *Circulation* **123**:2434–506.

Beckett NS, Peters R, Fletcher AE, et al. (2008). Treatment of hypertension in patients 80 years of age or older. *N Engl J Med* **358**:1887–98.

Joffres M, Falaschetti E, Gillespie C, et al. (2013). Hypertension prevalence, awareness, treatment and control in national surveys from England, the USA and Canada, and correlation with stroke and ischaemic heart disease mortality: a cross-sectional study. *BMJ Open* **3**:e003423.

Mancia G, Fagard R, Narkiewicz K, et al. (2013). 2013 ESH/ESC Guidelines for the management of arterial hypertension. The Task Force for the management of arterial hypertension of the European Society of Hypertension (ESH) and of the European Society of Cardiology (ESC). *Eur Heart J* **34**:2159–219.

Masoli JAH, Delgado J, Pilling L, et al. (2020). Blood pressure in frail older adults: associations with cardiovascular outcomes and all-cause mortality. *Age Ageing* **49**:807–13.

Reeve E, Jordan V, Thompson W, et al. (2020). Withdrawal of antihypertensive drugs in older people. *Cochrane Database Syst Rev* **6**:CD012572.

Saedon NI, Tan MP, Frith J (2020). The prevalence of orthostatic hypotension: a systematic review and meta-analysis. *J Gerontol A Biol Sci Med Sci* **75**:117–22.

Streit S, Poortvliet R, Gussekloo J (2018). Lower blood pressure during antihypertensive treatment is associated with higher all-cause mortality and accelerated cognitive decline in the oldest-old. Data from the Leiden 85-plus Study. *Age Ageing* **47**:545–50.

CHAPTER 24

Diagnosis and management of resistant hypertension

Fang-Fei Wei, Chen Liu, and Jan A. Staessen

KEY POINTS

* The prevalence of resistant hypertension among those receiving antihypertensive therapy is around 9–18%.

* A patient who is adherent to medication is considered to have resistant hypertension if their blood pressure is not controlled on maximally tolerated doses of three different classes of antihypertensive medications, including a diuretic.

* It is important to rule out secondary hypertension in patients with resistant hypertension.

* These patients are at high risk of cardiovascular complications.

* These patients may require the addition of mineralocorticoid antagonists, other diuretics, or centrally acting agents.

* Referral to a specialist hypertension clinic should be considered for further investigation and management.

24.1 Introduction

Hypertension is the predominant driver of cardiovascular disease and remains the leading cause of morbidity and mortality worldwide. Patients with resistant hypertension are at high risk of complications, particularly cardiovascular events. True resistant hypertension refers to a diagnosis of essential hypertension, with exclusion of all other potential causes of uncontrolled blood pressure, including secondary hypertension or pseudo-resistance due to poor adherence to antihypertensive therapy or the white coat effect. This chapter will focus on recent studies on the prevalence, associated risks, diagnosis, and management of resistant hypertension.

24.2 Epidemiology

Most epidemiological studies lack key elements for ascertaining the presence of resistant hypertension such as assessment of medication adherence and measurement of ambulatory blood pressure. The ideal design to estimate the prevalence of true resistant hypertension would be a large prospective cohort study of hypertensive patients with blood pressure control ascertained by ambulatory monitoring after forced titration up to the maximally tolerated doses of three different classes of antihypertensive medications, including a diuretic. To date, such a prospective study has not been published and the prevalence of resistant hypertension has been estimated using data from observational studies and outcome-based clinical trials.

24.2.1 Prevalence

The reported prevalence of resistant hypertension among patients who are receiving antihypertensive therapy is highly variable, ranging from 9% to 18%, because of divergent diagnostic approaches and non-exclusion of patients with pseudo-resistant hypertension. In a meta-analysis of 961,035 individuals, the prevalence of resistant hypertension was 13.7% (95% confidence interval (CI) 11.2–16.2) in 20 observational studies and 16.3% (95% CI 10.7–21.9) in four randomized trials; however, pseudo-resistance caused by suboptimal drug dosing, poor medication adherence, and the white coat effect could not be ruled out. Of 68,045 hypertensive patients enrolled in the Spanish Ambulatory Blood Pressure Monitoring Registry, 8295 (12.2%) had resistant hypertension defined as an increased office blood pressure whilst on treatment with three or more antihypertensive drugs, including a diuretic; however, the prevalence decreased to 5184 (7.6%) after those with white coat hypertension had been excluded. In the Ministero della Salute (MINISAL-SIIA) study, the investigators included 1284 patients with hypertension recruited from 47 Italian centres and excluded those with secondary or white coat hypertension. The prevalence of resistant hypertension among patients on stable drug therapy was 8.2% and increased 1.5-fold per 1 standard deviation (SD) increase in age and body mass index. However, accounting for adherence to lifestyle interventions, as indicated by a 24-hour urinary sodium excretion below 100 mmol and a normal body mass index, the prevalence of resistant hypertension was only 0.8%.

24.3 Associated risks

Resistant hypertension is associated with adverse health outcomes. In a retrospective analysis that included 205,750 patients in the United States with incident hypertension, the incidence of resistant hypertension within 1.5 years (median) from initial treatment was 1.9%, with a rate of 0.7 cases per 100 patient-years of follow-up. Patients with resistant hypertension had higher rates of baseline diabetes mellitus (17.7% versus 9.6%), compared with those with non-resistant hypertension. In multivariable-adjusted analyses, resistant hypertension was significantly associated with an increased risk of adverse cardiovascular outcomes over 3.8 years (median) (hazard ratio (HR) 1.47, 95% CI 1.33–1.62; p <0.001). Four subsequent studies strengthened the evidence for an association between resistant hypertension and cardiovascular events, but only one applied ambulatory blood pressure monitoring (ABPM) to exclude pseudo-resistance and none assessed treatment adherence. Among 1911 patients with treated hypertension, resistant hypertension was associated with an increased risk of cardiovascular events, compared to no history of resistant hypertension (HR 2.22, 95% CI 1.21–4.05). Among 14,684 patients enrolled in Antihypertensive and Lipid-Lowering Treatment to Prevent Heart Attack Trial (ALLHAT), apparent resistant hypertension was associated with an increased risk of all-cause mortality (HR 1.30, 95% CI 1.11–1.52), coronary heart disease (HR 1.44, 95% CI 1.18–1.76), heart failure (HR 1.88, 95% CI 1.52–2.34), stroke (HR 1.57, 95% CI 1.18–2.08), and end-stage renal disease (HR 1.95, 95% CI 1.11–3.41). Among 470,386 individuals with hypertension enrolled in the Kaiser Permanente Southern California healthcare programme, HRs were 1.06 for all-cause mortality (95% CI 1.03–1.08), 1.24 for ischaemic heart events (95% CI 1.20–1.28), 1.46 for congestive heart failure (95% 1.40–1.52), 1.14 for cerebrovascular accident (95% CI 1.10–1.19), and 1.32 for end-stage renal disease (95% CI 1.27–1.37).

24.4 Diagnosis

The first step in diagnosis is exclusion of secondary hypertension using the procedures that are outlined in current clinical practice guidelines.

24.4.1 Blood pressure measurement

ABPM is the current gold standard in blood pressure measurement. The time has come to revise the diagnosis of resistant hypertension by making ABPM a *condicio sine qua none*. Although the accuracy of ABPM can be limited by artefacts related to cuff size, movement, body position, short-term blood pressure variability, and interference with sleep, increased number of readings, absence of terminal digit preference and observer bias, and minimization of the white coat effect all contribute to the prognostic superiority of ambulatory blood pressure, compared with office blood pressure. A major contribution of ABPM to risk stratification is cross-classification between office and ambulatory blood pressures that enables true hypertension to be differentiated from white coat hypertension in untreated and treated patients.

24.4.2 Adherence

Poor drug adherence is a major problem in patients with resistant hypertension. Thus, drug adherence should always be assessed in these patients. Indirect methods to evaluate drug adherence, such as pill counts, patient interviews, self-reported drug use, heart rate on beta blockers, or activation of the renin–angiotensin–aldosterone system (RAAS) in response to treatment with angiotensin-converting enzyme (ACE) inhibitors or angiotensin I receptor blockers (ARBs), are vulnerable to biases or misclassification. Gold standard objective methods for assessing drug adherence include witnessed drug intake and measuring drugs or their metabolites in body fluids.

Poor adherence is an indicator of poor prognosis in patients with pseudo-resistant hypertension. The Italian Health Search/Thales database included 18,806 newly diagnosed hypertensive patients who were aged ≥35 years and initially free of cardiovascular disease. Six months after the index diagnosis, 8.1% were classified as having high adherence (proportion of days covered by filled prescriptions of ≥80%), 40.5% intermediate adherence (40–79%), and 51.4% low adherence (<40%). Over 4.6 years of follow-up, following statistical modelling and cumulative adjustments for confounders, high adherence was associated with a significantly reduced risk of acute cardiovascular events (HR 0.62, 95% CI 0.40–0.96; $p = 0.032$), compared with low adherence. However, >50% of patients with refractory hypertension remained non-compliant with medications when blood and urine samples were analysed to assess adherence. These data indicate that changes in adherence are a major potential confounder in trials of new treatment modalities for resistant hypertension.

24.5 Management

Renal sympathetic nerves have an important role in the pathogenesis of hypertension. Sympathetic nerve drive to the kidney is increased in patients with hypertension, particularly those with resistant hypertension. The approach to management of resistant hypertension, confirmed by ABPM and assessment of adherence, should be comprehensive and include lifestyle measures and management of risk factors such as dyslipidaemia, insulin resistance, and poor glycaemic control in patients with diabetes mellitus, in addition to pharmacological treatment.

24.5.1 Medical treatment

Optimizing pharmacological treatment of confirmed resistant hypertension is based on a few simple principles: (1) use of combinations of antihypertensive agents with different modes of action (blockers of the RAAS or a beta blocker with either a calcium channel blocker or a diuretic); (2) use of antihypertensive drugs with a long duration of action based on their molecular structure, so-called forgiving drugs, rather than on their extended-release dosage formulations; (3) titrating each drug to the highest dose that does not produce side effects; (4) including a diuretic in the drug combination; (5) once the right combination has been found by rotating through and combining drug classes, stimulating adherence by reducing the pill load with prescription of single-pill combination tablets, including two or three antihypertensive agents in adjustable doses; and (6) using aldosterone receptor antagonists or beta-1 blockers if not contraindicated.

Consistent with the notion that resistant hypertension is common among patients with primary hyperaldosteronism, mineralocorticoid receptor antagonists provide significant benefit in lowering blood pressure when added to existing multidrug regimens. The strongest evidence to support the use of mineralocorticoid receptor antagonists originates from the Prevention and Treatment of Hypertension with Algorithm based Therapy-2 (PATHWAY-2) trial (NCT 02369081). In this double-blind, placebo-controlled crossover trial, 335 patients were randomly assigned to sequential treatment with spironolactone, doxazosin, bisoprolol, and placebo. Eligibility criteria included age 18–79 years, seated clinic systolic pressure ≥140 mmHg (≥135 mmHg in diabetic patients), home systolic blood pressure (18 readings over 4 days) ≥130 mmHg, and treatment for at least 3 months with maximally tolerated doses of three antihypertensive drugs. Reduction in home systolic blood pressure with spironolactone averaged 8.7 mmHg (95% CI 7.7–9.7 mmHg) greater than with placebo, 4.0 mmHg (95% CI 3.0–5.0 mmHg) greater than with doxazosin, 4.5 mmHg (95% CI 3.5–5.5 mmHg) greater than with bisoprolol, and 4.3 mmHg (95% CI 3.4–5.1 mmHg) greater than the mean reduction with doxazosin and bisoprolol. Furthermore, spironolactone was the most effective blood pressure-lowering treatment throughout the distribution of plasma renin levels at baseline, but its margin of superiority and likelihood of being the best drug for the individual patient were greater at the lower than higher end of the plasma renin distribution. In only six of 285 patients on spironolactone, serum potassium levels exceeded 6.0 mmol/L on a single occasion, indicating that spironolactone can be administered without excessive risk of hyperkalaemia. However, the PATHWAY-2 results cannot be extrapolated to patients with treatment-resistant hypertension and estimated glomerular filtration rate (eGFR) <45 mL/min/1.73 m², because such patients were excluded from the trial. In a phase II multicentre, randomized, double-blind, placebo-controlled trial, 574 patients with resistant hypertension and chronic kidney disease (eGFR 25 to ≤45 mL/min/1.73 m²) were enrolled from 62 outpatient centres in ten countries and were randomly assigned to spironolactone, in addition to double-blind therapy with either placebo or patiromer. The investigators demonstrated that patiromer enabled more patients to continue treatment with spironolactone with less hyperkalaemia.

The most common adverse effect of spironolactone is breast tenderness, with or without breast enlargement, particularly in men. In this case, amiloride can be used as an alternative therapy. Amiloride antagonizes the epithelial sodium channel in the distal collecting duct of the kidney and functions as an indirect aldosterone antagonist. Moreover, arterial vasodilators, such as the potassium channel opener minoxidil or the selective endothelin type A antagonist darusantan, can also be considered for patients with resistant hypertension. However, some side effects, including fluid retention, oedema, and focal necrosis of the papillary heart muscle, limit their clinical application to patients in whom other medical treatment options have failed. Although mineralocorticoid receptor antagonists provide significant benefit in lowering blood pressure, clinical practice guidelines fall short in describing how blood pressure must be followed up in patients with resistant hypertension. After each optimization step of the drug regimen, ABPM should be repeated within 2–3 weeks to determine if adequate blood pressure reduction has been achieved. Once daytime and night-time blood pressures are controlled, ABPM must be repeated at 3- to 6-month intervals.

24.5.2 Device-based treatment

Potential options for device-based management of resistant hypertension include renal denervation, baroreflex activation therapy, arteriovenous anastomosis, and so on.

24.5.2.1 Renal denervation

In 2009, the investigators of renal sympathetic denervation in patients with treatment-resistant hypertension (SYMPLICITY HTN-1) trial demonstrated that percutaneous radiofrequency catheter-based renal sympathetic denervation was a feasible, effective, and safe intervention for treatment of resistant hypertension. Among 45 patients enrolled in this first-in-human study on treatment with 4.5 antihypertensive agents, systolic/diastolic blood pressures averaged 177/101 mmHg at entry and decreased by 27/17 mmHg at 12 months after renal denervation. Following this proof-of-concept study, the open SIMPLICITY HTN-2 trial randomly assigned 106 patients with resistant hypertension whose blood pressure on treatment with 5.2 drugs was 178/98 mmHg at entry and decreased by 32/12 mmHg in the denervation group, but did not change in control patients at 6 months' follow-up. In the subsequent single-blind, sham-controlled SYMPLICITY HTN-3 trial, the primary and secondary efficacy endpoints were changes in systolic blood pressure at 6 months, as evaluated by office blood pressure monitoring and 24-hour ABPM, respectively. Decreases in systolic blood pressure in the denervation group ($n = 364$), compared with controls ($n = 171$), were 14.1 mmHg versus 11.7 mmHg on office blood pressure monitoring and 6.8 mmHg versus 4.8 mmHg on ABPM, resulting in baseline-adjusted between-group differences of 2.4 mmHg (95% CI 2.1–6.9; $p = 0.26$) and 2.0 mmHg (95% CI −1.0 to 5.0; $p = 0.98$), respectively.

SYMPLICITY HTN-3 and other renal denervation trials with similarly disappointing results confirmed the safety, but not the efficacy, of the procedure. Notable exceptions to these disappointing results were the findings of the The Renal Denervation for Hypertension trial (DENERHTN) study and the AdenosINe Sestamibi Post-InfaRction Evaluation trial (INSPiRED) pilot trial. The DENERHTN trial demonstrated that approximately 6 mmHg greater decrease in 24-hour, daytime, and night-time systolic blood pressure at 6 months was in patients with resistant hypertension undergoing renal denervation together with standardized step-care antihypertensive treatment, compared with those on standardized step-care antihypertensive treatment alone. The INSPiRED pilot trial reported that the baseline-adjusted between-group differences in systolic/diastolic blood pressure were 19.5/10.4 mmHg for office blood pressure (7.6/2.2 mmHg in the control group versus −11.9/−8.2 mmHg in the renal denervation group; $p = 0.088$) and 22.4/13.1 mmHg for 24-hour blood pressure (0.7/0.3 mmHg in the control group versus −21.7/−12.8 mmHg in the renal denervation group; $p \leq 0.049$) at 6 months.

In view of the disappointing results of renal denervation in patients with treatment-resistant hypertension, subsequent trials have enrolled patients with untreated hypertension or treated mild hypertension and shortened follow-up from 6 to 3 months. The SPYRAL HTN-OFF MED study evaluated the effect of renal denervation on blood pressure in the absence of antihypertensive medications. Eligible patients were drug-naive (90%) or discontinued their antihypertensive drugs for 3–4 weeks prior to enrolment (10%) and had an office systolic blood pressure of 150–180 mmHg, a mean 24-hour ambulatory systolic blood pressure of 140–170 mmHg, and an office diastolic blood pressure of ≥90 mmHg. From baseline to 3-month follow-up, office and 24-hour ambulatory systolic and diastolic blood pressures decreased significantly (p ≤0.003) by 10.0/5.3 mmHg in the renal denervation group ($n = 38$) and by 5.5/4.8 mmHg in the control group ($n = 42$), resulting in mean baseline-adjusted differences of 7.7/4.9 mmHg (95% CI 1.5–14.0/−1.4 to 8.5 mmHg; p ≤0.016) on office measurement and 5.0/4.4 mmHg (95% CI 0.2–9.9/1.6–7.2 mmHg; p ≤0.041) on ambulatory monitoring. These data provide biological proof of principle that renal denervation, as done in this trial, lowers blood pressure in untreated patients with hypertension. The SPYRAL HTN-ON MED trial has a similar design to SPYRAL HTN OFF-MED but requires patients to be treated with a consistent triple-drug antihypertensive regimen prior to enrolment. At 6 months, the mean baseline-adjusted differences were 6.8/3.5 mmHg (1.1–12.5/0–7.0 mmHg) for office blood pressure and 7.4/4.1 mmHg (2.3–12.5/0.4–7.8 mmHg) for 24-hour blood pressure in favour of the renal denervation group (p ≤0.048). Fengler and colleagues compared the efficacy of radiofrequency and ultrasound endovascular renal denervation in patients with resistant hypertension. At 3 months, systolic daytime ambulatory blood pressure was more decreased in the ultrasound ablation group (−13.2 mmHg versus −6.5 mmHg; $p = 0.043$) than in the radiofrequency ablation group of the main renal artery.

24.5.3 Other device-based treatment

Activation of baroreceptors results in a reduction in blood pressure in patients with resistant hypertension by sympathetic inhibition. However, the evidence supporting carotid baroreceptor stimulation as a treatment modality in resistant hypertension remains weak. The most important limitations include the single-arm, unblind design of most previous studies, variable follow-up duration, use of office monitoring, rather than 24-hour ABPM, and lack of reliable data on adherence.

The novel arteriovenous ROX Coupler (ROX Medical, San Clemente, CA, USA) reduces blood pressure by adding a low-resistance, high-compliance venous segment to the central arterial tree. An open-label, randomized trial assessed the efficacy of this device in 83 patients with uncontrolled hypertension. However, the acute and long-term safety of the approach remains to be proven.

24.6 Conclusion

Once a diagnosis of resistant hypertension is confirmed, optimization of drug treatment and ensuring adherence to medications remain the cornerstone of its management. For now, device treatment should remain the last resort in adherent and truly resistant patients with severe hypertension, in whom all other efforts to reduce blood pressure have failed and should only be offered to patients within the context of clinical research in highly skilled tertiary referral centres. However, in non-adherent patients, educational measures, behavioural interventions, and eHealth interventions would probably be a better strategy. Future research should focus on a better understanding of the intrinsic (in the patients) and extrinsic (e.g. environmental stressors) mechanisms that contribute to an adherent patient's lack of responsiveness to blood pressure-lowering drugs.

KEY REFERENCES

Achelrod D, Wenzel U, Frey S (2015). Systematic review and meta-analysis of the prevalence of resistant hypertension in treated hypertensive populations. *Am J Hypertens* **28**:355–61.

Calhoun DA, Jones D, Textor S, et al. (2008). Resistant hypertension: diagnosis, evaluation, and treatment. A scientific statement from the American Heart Association Professional Education Committee of the Council for High Blood Pressure Research. *Hypertension* **51**:1403–19.

de Jager RL, de Beus E, Beeftink MM, et al. (2017). The impact of medication adherence on the effect of renal denervation. The SYMPATHY trial. *Hypertension* **69**:678–84.

Fengler k, Rommel K, Blazek S, et al. (2019). A three-arm randomized trial of different renal denervation devices and techniques in patients with resistant hypertension (RADIOSOUND-HTN) circulation **139**:590–600.

Galletti F, Barbato A (2016). Prevalence and determinants of resistant hypertension in a sample of patients followed in Italian hypertension centers: results from the MINISAL-SIIA study program. *J Hum Hypertens* **30**:703–8.

GBD 2016 Risk Factors Collaborators (2017). Global, regional, and national comparative risk assessment of 84 behavioural, environmental and occupational, and metabolic risks or clusters of risks, 1990–2016: a systematic analysis for the Global Burden of Disease Study 2016. *Lancet* **390**:1345–422.

Heusser K, Tank J, Engeli S, et al. (2020). Carotid baroreceptor stimulation, sympathetic activity, baroreflex function, and blood pressure in hypertensive patients. *Hypertension* **55**:619–26.

Krum H, Schlaich M, Whitbourn R, et al. (2009). Catheter-based renal sympathetic denervation for resistant hypertension: a multicentre safety and proof-of-principle cohort study. *Lancet* **373**:1275–81.

Persu A, Renkin J, Thijs L, Staessen JA (2012). Renal denervation: ultima ratio or standard in treatment-resistant hypertension. *Hypertension* **60**:596–606.

Sim JJ, Bhandari SK, Shi J, et al. (2015). Comparative risk of renal, cardiovascular, and mortality outcomes in controlled, uncontrolled resistant, and non-resistant hypertension. *Kidney Int* **88**:622–32.

Townsend RR, Mahfoud F, Kandzari DE, et al. (2017). Catheter-based renal denervation in patients with uncontrolled hypertension in the absence of antihypertensive medications (SPYRAL HTN-OFF MED): a randomised, sham-controlled, proof-of-concept trial. *Lancet* **390**:2160–70.

Tsioufis C, Kordalis A, Flessas D, et al. (2011). Pathophysiology of resistant hypertension: role of the sympathetic nervous system. *Int J Hypertens* **2011**:642416.

CHAPTER 25

Hypertension in patients with diabetes mellitus

Daniel J. Cuthbertson

KEY POINTS

* Hypertension frequently coexists with diabetes, increasing the risk of both macrovascular and microvascular complications.
* Clinical trials have demonstrated the effectiveness of blood pressure lowering in reducing these diabetes complications.
* Multiple pathophysiological mechanisms explain this coexistence, including insulin resistance and hyperinsulinaemia, activation of the renin–angiotensin system, plasma volume expansion, and increased arterial stiffness.
* Effective management of diabetes should target optimal blood pressure and lipid management with individualized glycaemic control.
* Use of angiotensin-converting enzyme inhibitors or angiotensin receptor blockers should be used as first-line therapy for blood pressure lowering, as monotherapy or in combinations, to prevent or reduce the burden of atherosclerotic cardiovascular disease, heart failure, and microvascular complications.

25.1 Introduction

Globally, we are experiencing a pandemic of overweight and obesity, with a parallel rise in the number of people with diabetes. In 2014, according to the World Health Organization, there were an estimated 422 million people with diabetes, with the prevalence rising more rapidly in low- and middle-income countries, reaching 642 million by 2040. Around 95% of these people with diabetes will have type 2 diabetes (T2D), most commonly linked with abdominal obesity, causing insulin resistance and hyperinsulinaemia. Type 1 diabetes has a very distinct pathophysiology secondary to autoimmune mediated pancreatic beta cell destruction and absolute insulin deficiency.

Diabetes mellitus is characterized by micro- and macrovascular complications, which contribute significantly to associated morbidity and mortality and associated lost years of life expectancy. Such complications include macrovascular or atherosclerotic cardiovascular disease (ASCVD) (stroke, coronary artery disease, and peripheral vascular disease), heart failure, and microvascular complications (including retinopathy, nephropathy, and neuropathy). Diabetes increases the risk of cardiovascular disease (CVD) and stroke by 2- to 4-fold above that for a person without diabetes. The Multiple Risk Factor Interventional Trial (MRFIT) demonstrated a persisting residual increased risk with diabetes, even after adjusting for age and other cardiovascular risk factors such as hypertension, smoking, and hyperlipidaemia. Similarly, a prospective Finnish study highlighted the risk of coronary artery-related death was comparable in patients with diabetes and no prior history of myocardial infarction to those without diabetes but with prior myocardial infarction.

25.2 Definition of hypertension

Hypertension is defined as a sustained blood pressure of ≥140/90 mmHg, according to various definitions, although some guidelines have suggested lower blood pressure recordings. This is discussed in detail in other chapters of this book.

25.3 Epidemiology/prevalence of diabetes and hypertension

Excluding obesity, arterial hypertension and T2D account for the most prevalent cardiovascular risk factors in the global population. However, whilst the prevalence of T2D is continuing to increase, the prevalence, awareness, and treatment of hypertension in higher-income countries have reduced over the last few decades. Although hypertension is more common in patients with diabetes, its prevalence in diabetes is influenced by various factors, including age, sex, ethnicity, and body mass index of the patient, the type and duration of diabetes, the associated glycaemic control (HbA1c level), and whether there is underlying chronic kidney disease (CKD). Hypertension is more common with advancing age and in people of black African or African-Caribbean origin.

Hypertension prevalence rates in people with T2D approach 80% in many European countries; its high prevalence reflects the typical clustering of cardiometabolic risk factors (abdominal obesity, dyslipidaemia, hypertension, etc.) seen as a component of the metabolic syndrome. In contrast, hypertension prevalence rates in people with T1D are much lower, with the incidence rising from around 5% at 10 years to about 30% at 20 years; its development may represent the onset of diabetic nephropathy.

There is a robust bidirectional relationship between hypertension and T2D, but the causality between the two conditions has hitherto been unclear. A recent Mendelian randomization analysis of >300,000 people without baseline CVD or T2D from the UK Biobank has shown that whilst T2D is causal for hypertension development, the reverse does not apply (i.e. hypertension is not causal for T2D). Genetically predisposed T2D was related to a 7% increased risk of hypertension, associated with a 0.67 mmHg higher systolic blood pressure (BP), with no difference in diastolic BP.

25.4 Prognostic impact of hypertension in diabetes

Hypertension is a major risk factor for major adverse cardiovascular events, CKD, cognitive decline, and premature death. However, the coexistence of hypertension with both type 1 diabetes and T2D substantially worsens clinical outcomes, increasing the risk of both macrovascular or atherosclerotic CVD (stroke, coronary artery disease, and peripheral vascular disease), heart failure, and microvascular complications (including retinopathy, nephropathy, and neuropathy).

In the Hypertension in Diabetes Study, patients with hypertension and T2D, compared to non-hypertensive patients with T2D, had higher rates of CVD death, ischaemic heart disease, amputation, and stroke, independent of other risk factors. This higher rate of diabetes-related complications, attributable to coexisting hypertension, has been shown in other studies. In type 1 diabetes, the strongest relationship with outcomes is probably related to evolution of proteinuria and progression of CKD.

25.5 Pathophysiology of hypertension in diabetes

There are multiple pathophysiological mechanisms that explain this coexistence of hypertension and diabetes with insulin resistance and hyperinsulinaemia, either compensatory hyperinsulinaemia or due to exogenous insulin administration.

- Insulin usually has vasodilatory activity, mediated by nitric oxide, and thus loss of this vasodilatory capacity may increase systemic BP,
- Insulin increases sympathetic activity and promotes sodium and water reabsorption at the distal tubule, promoting volume expansion,
- Hyperglycaemia-induced increase in filtered glucose load leads to increased proximal tubular glucose reabsorption (via sodium–glucose co-transporters), resulting in a parallel rise in sodium reabsorption,
- Increased arterial stiffness due to increased protein glycation, and
- Activation of the renin–angiotensin system.

25.6 Recommendations

Broadly speaking, there are several general principles regarding BP management in diabetes that should be considered.

25.6.1 Measurement of blood pressure

Addressing cardiovascular risk factors, especially BP and cholesterol, is now part of routine diabetes care. Measurement of BP at every clinic visit is recommended. All patients with elevated BP should have confirmatory/multiple readings on a separate day within 1 month due to considerable normal variation of BP. Domiciliary BP monitoring is also recommended to exclude white coat hypertension. The American Diabetes Association (ADA) position statement recommends that most adults with diabetes achieve BP of <140/90 mmHg.

25.6.2 Assess target organ/end-organ damage

Damage to organs such as the heart (e.g. left ventricular hypertrophy), kidneys (increased urine albumin:creatinine ratio (UACR) or CKD with evidence of reductions in estimated glomerular filtration rate (eGFR) or increased serum creatinine)), or eyes (hypertensive retinopathy) should be carefully assessed.

25.6.3 Consider cardiovascular risk

Cardiovascular risk or assessment of ASCVD is critical and will influence choice and aggressiveness of treatment targets for glucose and blood pressure lowering.

25.7 Evidence for impact of blood pressure lowering on outcomes in diabetes

Randomized clinical trials have demonstrated the effectiveness of aggressive treatment of hypertension and BP lowering in reducing these diabetes complications and specifically in reducing associated cardiovascular morbidity and mortality.

25.7.1 UK Prospective Diabetes Study

In the UK Prospective Diabetes Study (UKPDS) blood pressure study, 1148 people were randomized to tight BP control (n = 758) or less tight BP control (n = 390); final mean difference between the two groups was 10/5 mmHg (154/87 mmHg versus 144/82 mmHg). Treatment was with the beta blocker atenolol or the ACE inhibitor captopril. Over 9 years, those assigned to the tight BP control arm had significant reductions in morbidity and mortality:

- 32% in deaths related to diabetes (6–51%) (p = 0.019)
- 24% in diabetes-related endpoints (95% confidence interval (CI) 8–38%) (p = 0.0046)
- 44% reduction in fatal and non-fatal stroke (11–65%) (p = 0.013)
- 56% reduction in congestive cardiac failure
- 37% in microvascular endpoints (11–56%) (p = 0.0092), predominantly due to reduced risk of retinal photocoagulation.

25.7.2 Hypertension Optimal Treatment

Further evidence of benefit of BP lowering in T2D comes from the Hypertension Optimal Treatment (HOT) study of 18,790 people (1500 people with T2D) with hypertension, randomized into three groups, aiming to achieve diastolic BPs of

≤90, ≤85, or ≤80 mmHg. Relative risk reduction of 51% was observed in cardiovascular morbidity and mortality with tightest versus least tight control.

25.7.3 Steno-2 intervention study

This study of 160 people with T2D and microalbuminuria, a population at significant risk of CVD, randomized 80 people to conventional treatment and 80 to intensive treatment aiming to treat all cardiovascular risk factors simultaneously. For those who received intensive treatment, the aim was: to reduce cholesterol to ≤4.5 mmol/L, HbA1c level to ≤48 mmol/mol (≤6.5%), and BP to ≤130/80 mmHg; to prescribe aspirin; and for participants to stop smoking. After a mean follow-up of 7.8 years, there was a significant reduction in both macro- and microvascular disease endpoints by approximately 50%.

An observational follow-up of the Steno-2 study after 13.3 years reported the benefits of tight BP control (with strict glycaemic control and lipid lowering) in at-risk people with T2D continued. Twenty-four people in the intensive treatment group had died, compared to 40 in the standard treatment group, and intensive therapy was associated with a lower risk of death from cardiovascular causes (hazard ratio 0.43, 95% CI 0.19–0.94; $p = 0.04$) and of cardiovascular events (hazard ratio 0.41, 95% CI 0.25–0.67; $p < 0.001$).

25.7.4 Systematic review and meta-analysis

A recent systematic review and meta-analysis of trials that either reported diabetic subgroups or included only diabetic patients examined the impact of BP control. Forty trials, involving 100,354 participants, were included—every 10 mmHg reduction in BP was associated with significant reductions in micro- and macrovascular outcomes, including heart failure and total mortality.

25.8 Optimal blood pressure treatment target

The goal of treatment is BP <140/80 mmHg, with a more aggressive goal of <130/80 mmHg in patients with a higher risk of CVD. Meta-analyses consistently show that treating patients with a baseline BP of ≥140 mmHg to targets of <140 mmHg is beneficial, whilst more intensive targets may offer additional (though probably less robust) benefits. The Action to Control Cardiovascular Risk in Diabetes (ACCORD) BP results suggest that BP targets more intensive than <140/90 mmHg are not likely to improve cardiovascular outcomes among most people with T2D.

Guidance from the National Institute for Health and Care Excellence (NICE) states that, with respect to type 1 diabetes, intervention levels for recommending BP management should be 135/85 mmHg unless the adult with type 1 diabetes has albuminuria or two or more features of the metabolic syndrome, in which case it should be 130/80 mmHg.

25.9 Treatment of blood pressure

25.9.1 Lifestyle modification

Lifestyle modification includes weight loss, dietary sodium restriction and a healthy balanced diet, regular exercise, avoiding excess ethanol ingestion, and smoking cessation.

25.9.2 Antihypertensive medication

25.9.2.1 Principles of effective use

Single antihypertensive drug use may be inadequate, particularly depending on the initial BP, and stepwise titration is needed until adequate BP control is achieved. Drugs should be titrated carefully to the maximum (tolerated) dose, and compliance/adherence reinforced. Multiple drug use is usually necessary. Various factors influence response to pharmacological treatment.

BP targets should be individualized through shared decision-making that addresses cardiovascular risk and potential adverse effects of antihypertensive drugs, and considers patient preferences.

25.9.2.2 Choice of agent

Initial treatment should include drug classes demonstrated to reduce cardiovascular events in patients with T2D: ACE inhibitors, angiotensin receptor blockers (ARBs), thiazide-like diuretics, or dihydropyridine calcium channel blockers (CCBs).

The recommendation is to start with an ACE inhibitor or ARB if side effects of ACE inhibitor therapy (usually cough) mean that they cannot be tolerated. ACE inhibitors/ARBs reduce the risk of progressive kidney disease in patients with albuminuria (UACR ≥30 mg/g creatinine).

If full-dose ACE/ARB therapy does not control BP to the recommended targets, NICE recommends adding a CCB or diuretic (usually a thiazide or thiazide-related diuretic).

People of African-Caribbean descent may be relatively resistant to ACE inhibitor monotherapy, and so NICE recommends using an ACE inhibitor plus either a diuretic or a CCB as initial therapy.

If dual therapy with an ACE inhibitor plus a diuretic, or an ACE inhibitor plus a CCB, does not control BP to target, the agent not used out of the three—CCB or diuretic—should be added to give a triple-agent regimen. If a fourth agent is required, NICE recommends using an alpha blocker, a beta blocker, or a potassium-sparing diuretic.

25.9.2.3 Glucose-lowering treatment

Thiazolidinediones, dipeptidyl peptidase 4 (DPP-4) inhibitors, glucagon-like peptide 1 (GLP-1) receptor agonists, and sodium–glucose co-transporter-2 (SGLT-2) inhibitors have all been associated with a decrease in BP.

25.10 Conclusion

Hypertension is a major modifiable risk factor in patients with type 1 diabetes and T2D, increasing the risk of macrovascular CVD or ASCVD, heart failure, and microvascular complications. Multiple pathophysiological mechanisms underlie this coexistence, including insulin resistance and hyperinsulinaemia, activation of the renin–angiotensin system, plasma volume expansion, and increased arterial stiffness. Fortunately, the results of many randomized clinical trials have demonstrated the effectiveness of BP lowering in reducing the burden of these diabetes complications. Effective management of diabetes should target optimal BP control, alongside effective lipid management and individualized glycaemic control.

KEY REFERENCES

[No authors listed] (1993). Hypertension in Diabetes Study (HDS): II. Increased risk of cardiovascular complications in hypertensive type 2 diabetic patients. *J Hypertens* 11.319–25.

de Boer IH, Bangalore S, Benetos A, *et al.* (2017). Diabetes and hypertension: a position statement by the American Diabetes Association. *Diabetes Care* 40:1273–84.

Emdin CA, Rahimi K, Neal B, Callender T, Perkovic V, Patel A (2015). Blood pressure lowering in type 2 diabetes: a systematic review and meta-analysis. *JAMA* 313:603–15.

Gaede P, Lund-Andersen H, Parving HH, Pedersen O (2008). Effect of a multifactorial intervention on mortality in type 2 diabetes. *N Engl J Med* 358:580–91.

Gaede P, Vedel P, Larsen N, Jensen GV, Parving HH, Pedersen O (2003). Multifactorial intervention and cardiovascular disease in patients with type 2 diabetes. *N Engl J Med* 348:383–93.

Hansson L, Zanchetti A, Carruthers SG, *et al.* (1998). Effects of intensive blood-pressure lowering and low-dose aspirin in patients with hypertension: principal results of the Hypertension Optimal Treatment (HOT) randomised trial. HOT Study Group. *Lancet* 351:1755–62.

Mehler PS, Jeffers BW, Estacio R, Schrier RW (1997). Associations of hypertension and complications in non-insulin-dependent diabetes mellitus. *Am J Hypertens* 10:152–61.

Mills KT, Bundy JD, Kelly TN, *et al.* (2016). Global disparities of hypertension prevalence and control: a systematic analysis of population-based studies from 90 countries. *Circulation* 134:441–50.

Ogurtsova K, da Rocha Fernandes JD, Huang Y, *et al.* (2017). IDF Diabetes Atlas: global estimates for the prevalence of diabetes for 2015 and 2040. *Diabetes Res Clin Pract* 128:40–50.

Sun D, Zhou T, Heianza Y, *et al.* (2019). Type 2 diabetes and hypertension. *Circulation Res* 124:930–7.

UK Prospective Diabetes Study Group (1998). Tight blood pressure control and risk of macrovascular and microvascular complications in type 2 diabetes: UKPDS 38. UK Prospective Diabetes Study Group. *BMJ* 317:703–13.

Index

For the benefit of digital users, indexed terms that span two pages (e.g., 52–53) may, on occasion, appear on only one of those pages.

Tables, figures, and boxes are indicated by t, f, and b following the page number